Help
Your
Self

Help Your Self

Self

THE NEW RULES FOR WELLNESS

MEREDITH BAIRD
& KATERINA SCHNEIDER

Abrams, New York

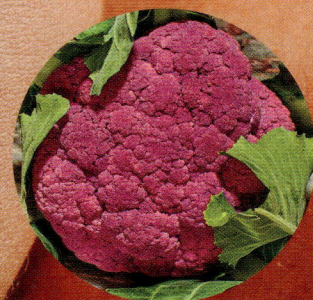

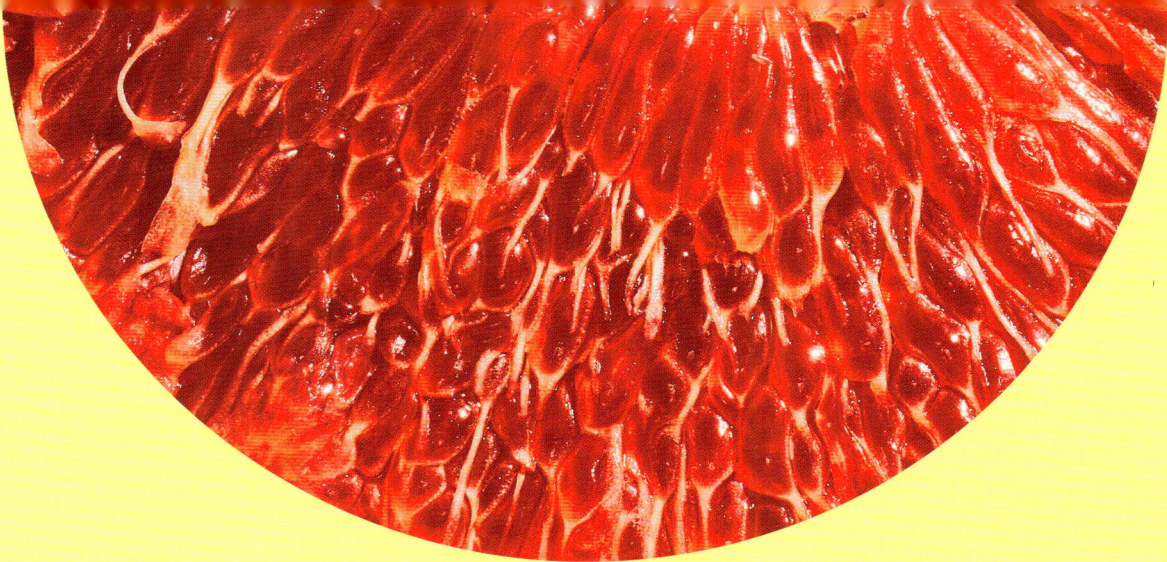

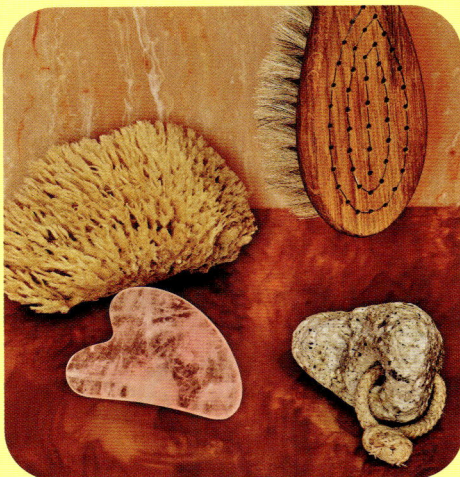

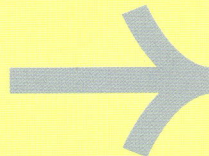

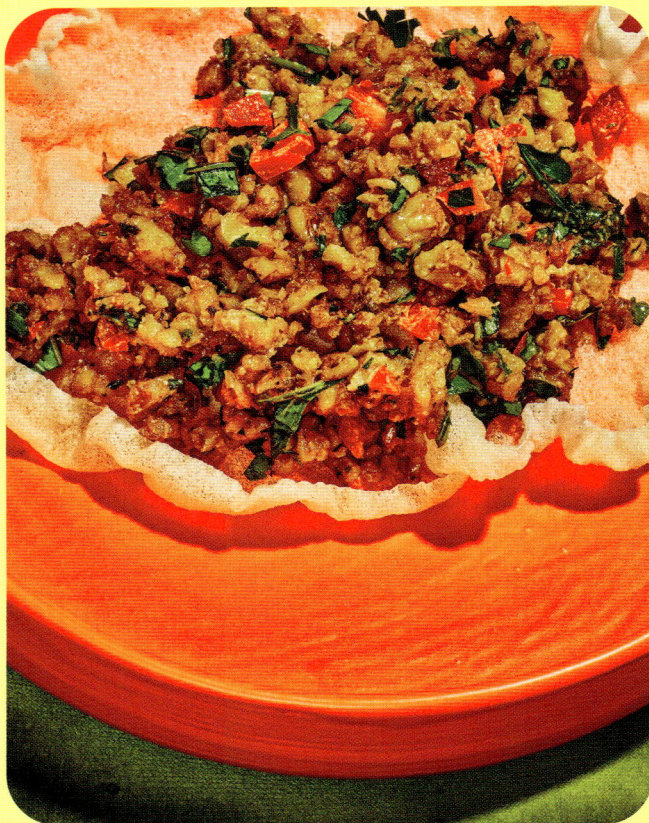

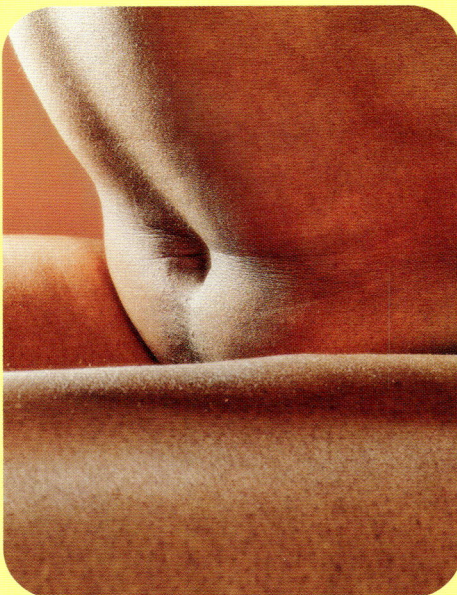

CONTENTS

Help
your

There is a lot on our plates, and that doesn't even include dinner. As the pursuit of wellness reaches a fever pitch, the lines between fact and fringe have blurred. We know what we want: clear, accurate information that empowers us to make healthy choices for ourselves and our families. But it feels like wellness has become a full-time job, forcing us to become obsessive researchers and pseudoscientists. Who has time for that?

We get it, and we're here to help. As two wellness industry insiders, entrepreneurs, and busy moms, we want to make this easy for you. Our mission with this book is to tune out the noise, dismantle the half-truths, and separate fact from fiction when it comes to wellness. We've spent our careers unearthing the latest in health research, and in the pages that follow, we're going to settle the score on what's science and what's ceremony when it comes to the health trends that are floating around out there—all in the name of empowering you to *help your self.*

Self

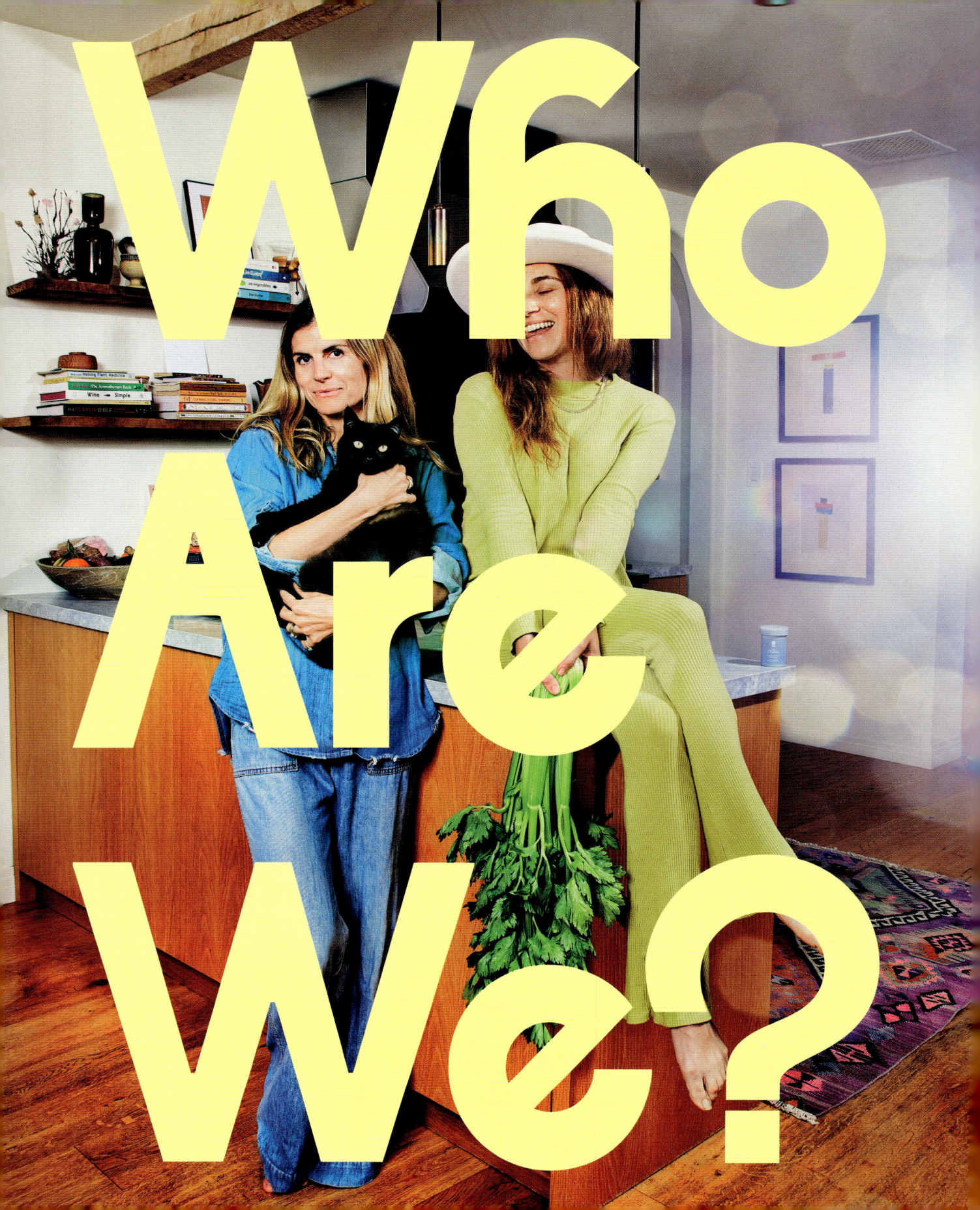

Who Are We?

Every friendship has a foundation, and ours is built on refusing to settle.

When Kat got pregnant and couldn't find a prenatal vitamin with ingredients she trusted, she assembled a world-class scientific team to create one. The result? Her health technology company, Ritual, which produces prenatal vitamins made from the highest-quality ingredients.

When Meredith was handed a prescription for her psoriasis diagnosis, she intuitively knew there had to be another way. Returning to her roots in the kitchen, she began experimenting with the topical power of plants, and after months of trial and error (not to mention profound skin shifts), Nucifera—her multipurpose vegan skin care line—was born.

The real magic happened when we first met, and Kat was looking for a recipe developer to help her with what eventually became Ritual vitamins.

As new moms, we connected over our shared values, and we were both deeply invested in a deeper understanding of health.

We debated the merits of stainless steel versus glass cookware, shared tips for making our own seed milks, and discussed the pros and cons of different water filters—and we immediately bonded over our health-geeky tendencies. We covered a lot of ground, from clever ways to feed our kids vegetables (you know, picky-eater hacks) to conversations about mental health, marriage, and balancing life while running our businesses. Along the way, a lifelong friendship was born.

When it comes to health and wellness techniques, we have been there, done that. And in this book, from the esoteric to the mainstream, we're going to spell it all out for you—so that you can skip the woo-woo and go straight to, "Wait. This actually works."

There's no question that we are more focused on our health today than at any time in history. And that's a good thing—to a point. As a result, the wellness industry is booming, having surpassed a value of $5 trillion in 2020, with plant-based food sales increasing more than 45 percent since 2021. This translates to a limitless—and overwhelming—range of options to navigate. But we're here to show you that all of this can be easier (and more enjoyable) than you think. Making good health choices doesn't have to mean spending a ton of time or breaking the bank.

So, let's get after it →

● HOW TO USE THIS BOOK

We recommend reading this book from start to finish, keeping in mind that there is a lot of information to absorb in these pages. Don't feel like you have to master it all at once or throw out everything in your pantry or medicine cabinet. Think more in terms of making gradual, sustainable changes to your daily habits, incorporating what feels right to you, and disregarding what doesn't.

What we hope you'll take away is a greater understanding of how our bodily systems and responses work together, and that better health is often about finding a rhythm. If your stress is unregulated, it might be helpful to look at your gut health or sleeping patterns, and how hydrating properly can help improve your gut health and so on. Culturally we are taught to look at the symptom as an isolated experience instead of looking at everything holistically—but it is imperative to look at the whole picture. Starting to understand the rhythmic way our bodies work can be deeply rewarding and initiate a chain of positive health benefits.

In some chapters, you will see that we include a section called "The Routine," where we spotlight our favorite daily rituals. We don't want you to feel pressure to recreate these routines if they don't work for your lifestyle. They are meant to be aspirational and inspirational, and you can tailor them as you see fit. The reward at the end of each chapter is some of our favorite easy and delicious plant-based recipes to add to your repertoire.

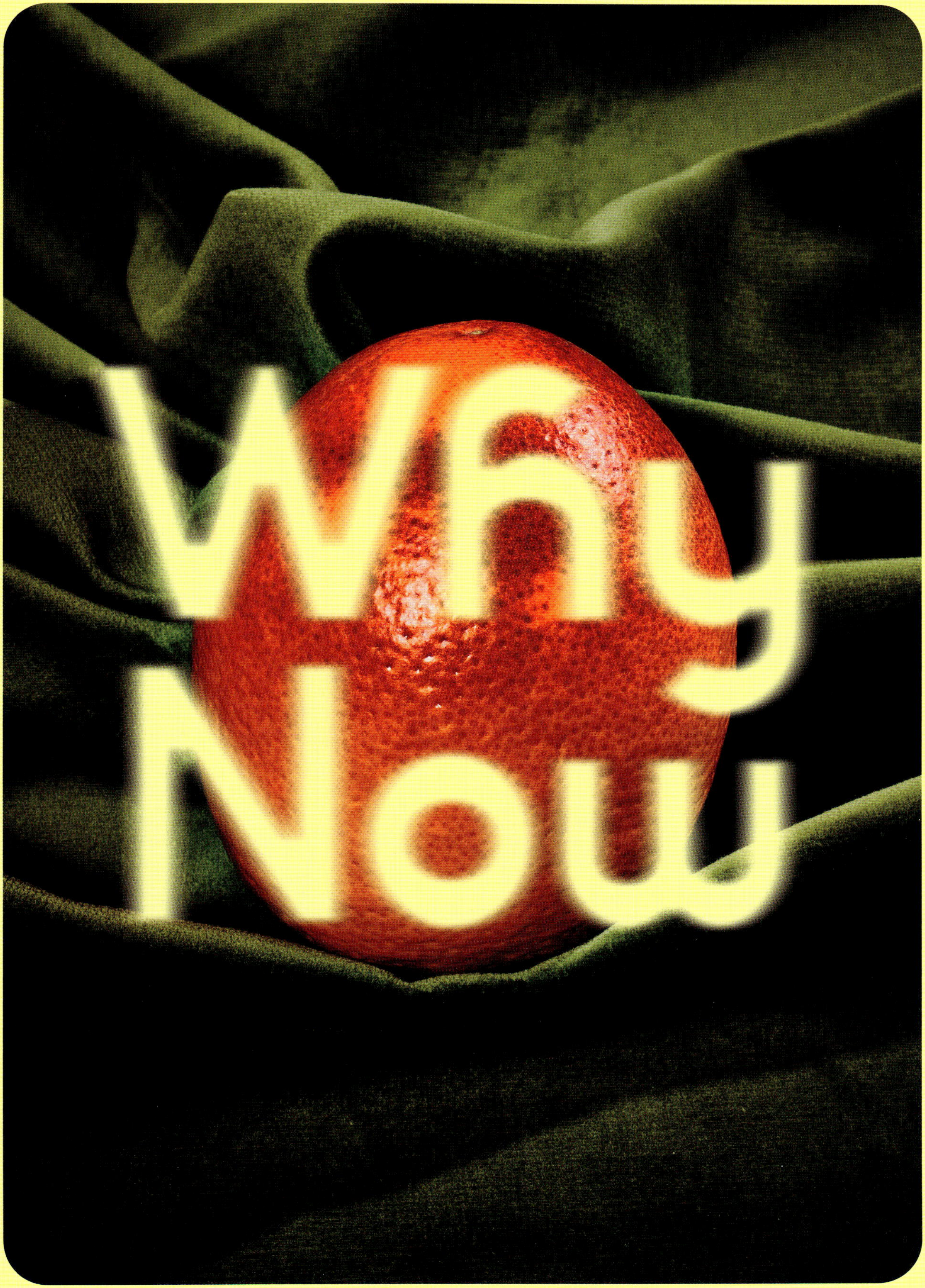
Why
Now

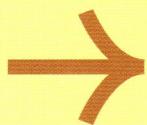
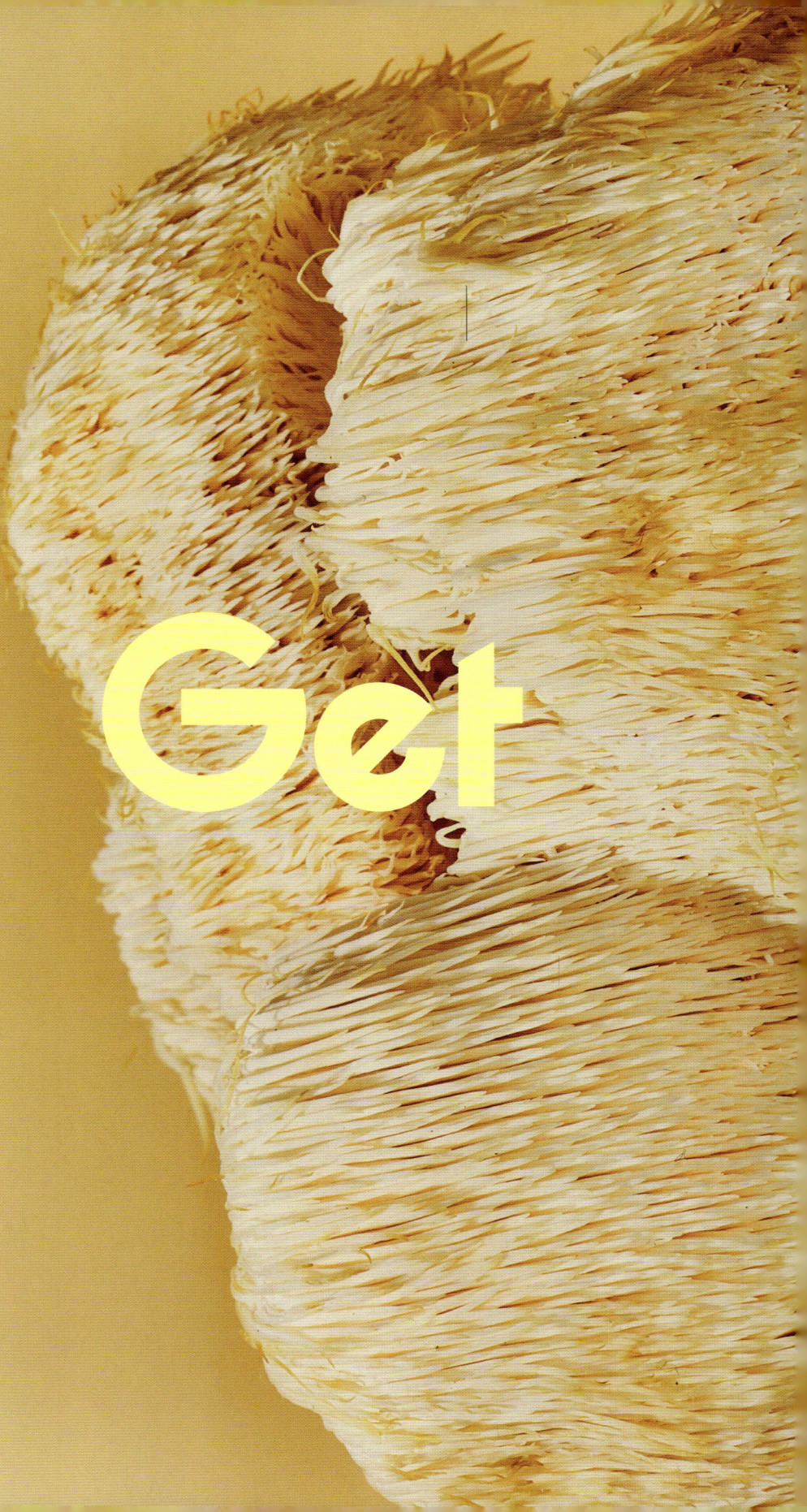

Get

Started

"

I didn't become a plant-based eater until ten-plus years ago. My body always craved vegetables, and I never felt well eating meat, but because I grew up in an Eastern European family (from Ukraine), it was always expected that meat was the centerpiece of our meals.

That changed for me and for my family when we started to expand our worldview with holistic health and macrobiotics. When I was in high school, my parents bought a Norman Walker juicer, and I started telling everyone that if their juice wasn't pressed, it wasn't good enough. Later, my mom became a macrobiotic foods practitioner and primarily cooked for us that way at home. After a terrible breakup in my twenties, I went deep into my yoga practice and decided to give up meat. My yoga guru said, "The energy of the animals you eat will stay with you for the rest of your life." If the health benefits of giving up dairy and meat weren't enough, the spiritual and psychological plus the animal rights aspects certainly had a profound impact on my decision to stop.

Almost immediately, my acne cleared up, and I started feeling lighter and happier. I learned and experimented so much in those early years. Becoming pregnant with my first child, and wanting to nourish myself as deeply and efficiently as possible, then led to my decision to start my company, Ritual. This made me dive deeper into the science of plant-based eating and embrace all the alternative health practices that I had been exposed to throughout my life.

In many ways, this book is the culmination of the two sides of my health life: the factual, clinically researched side that centers around Ritual, and the intuitive, experimental side that I grew up with.

—KAT

This is the chapter to get you inspired. We're going to cover the basics of kickstarting your wellness—from using nontoxic cookware at home to embracing the new food pyramid. Establishing a solid foundation with these basics is essential, before you move on to more targeted wellness protocols and products.

The Power of Plant-Based

Many of us have been fooled into thinking that eating a healthy diet must be complicated, expensive, and time consuming. However, when we look at the world's healthiest and longest-living populations, such as those living in the Blue Zones (regions of the world where people live longer, healthier lives compared with the global average), we see they eat simply, locally, and inexpensively—with much less access to choice than we have in the average grocery store. The foundational foods in these cultures are whole grains and beans or legumes, local and seasonal vegetables and fruit, and unprocessed meat and dairy eaten in moderation, although these foods are rarely eliminated completely. The key difference between the standard American diet and diets found in these cultures is less reliance on processed foods, including refined grains and carbs.

Research shows that following a primarily whole foods, plant-based diet, in which meat and dairy are consumed in moderation, has significant health benefits, including improved digestion, reduced risk of chronic disease, weight management, improvements in heart health, and the list goes on. We aren't advocating for the elimination of any food group. Eating plant-based doesn't mean avoiding animal products entirely—it means eating a diverse range of foods that come from the earth (vegetables, fruits, whole grains, legumes). It means limiting the use of refined oils, added sugars, and anything processed. It means eating whole foods that are rich in fiber, vitamins, minerals, and antioxidants. And getting excited about plants! Keep in mind that just because a packaged snack says "organic" or "vegan" doesn't mean it's good for you.

Many of us have the impression that eating a plant-based diet will be prohibitively expensive, or that plant-based ingredients are hard to find in your average grocery store. In truth, while certain plant-based specialty products may be pricey, staples like beans, grains, veggies, and fruits are often more affordable than their animal-based counterparts. Eating plant-based does not have to be expensive, complicated, or intimidating in any way. We want to liberate you from these misconceptions so that you can Help Your Self to eat and feel better.

In this chapter, we will break down the basics on how to pull together an affordable, nutritionally complete, plant-based meal. We'll also share a delicious foundational recipe for making your own homemade nut milk as a cheaper and healthier alternative to buying commercial-brand nut milk (which is often loaded with additives and preservatives).

Principles for Getting Started

As you start this journey, these are a few principles
to embrace that will help you along the way.

→ Be prepared

True wellness starts with preparation, from stocking your home and pantry with healthy ingredients, to mastering a few simple recipes (like those in this chapter) so that you can pull together a quick and easy meal. This principle also includes meal prep tricks like washing and chopping veggies on Sunday for the week ahead and investing in green, nontoxic cookware.

→ Listen to your body

We can point to scientific data and research studies to show you why something is good for you, but ultimately, you know your body best. If a health trend doesn't feel right to you, skip it and go with your gut. This is why we always look to time-honored traditions that are grounded and seasonal, and tend to approach trends with caution.

→ Make it a ritual

If you can't make something into a ritual that you'll look forward to doing each day, you're not going to stick with it, and it's not going to have a meaningful impact on your health. Fad diets, elaborate supplement routines, overly intense workout schedules—these things come and go. Instead, focus on building habits that you will be able to maintain. Health is not what you do perfectly every single day; it is the culmination of what you do most often.

→ Live simply

As we've mentioned, we are inspired by those populations within the world's Blue Zones, who regularly live to their eighties, nineties, and even upwards of one hundred years old. These people take a pura vida—pure life—approach to wellness, which includes drinking more water (and eating hydrating foods), eating for enjoyment, walking more, and spending time together in community. If we don't master these foundational basics, it's not worth investing in the next layer of wellness concepts.

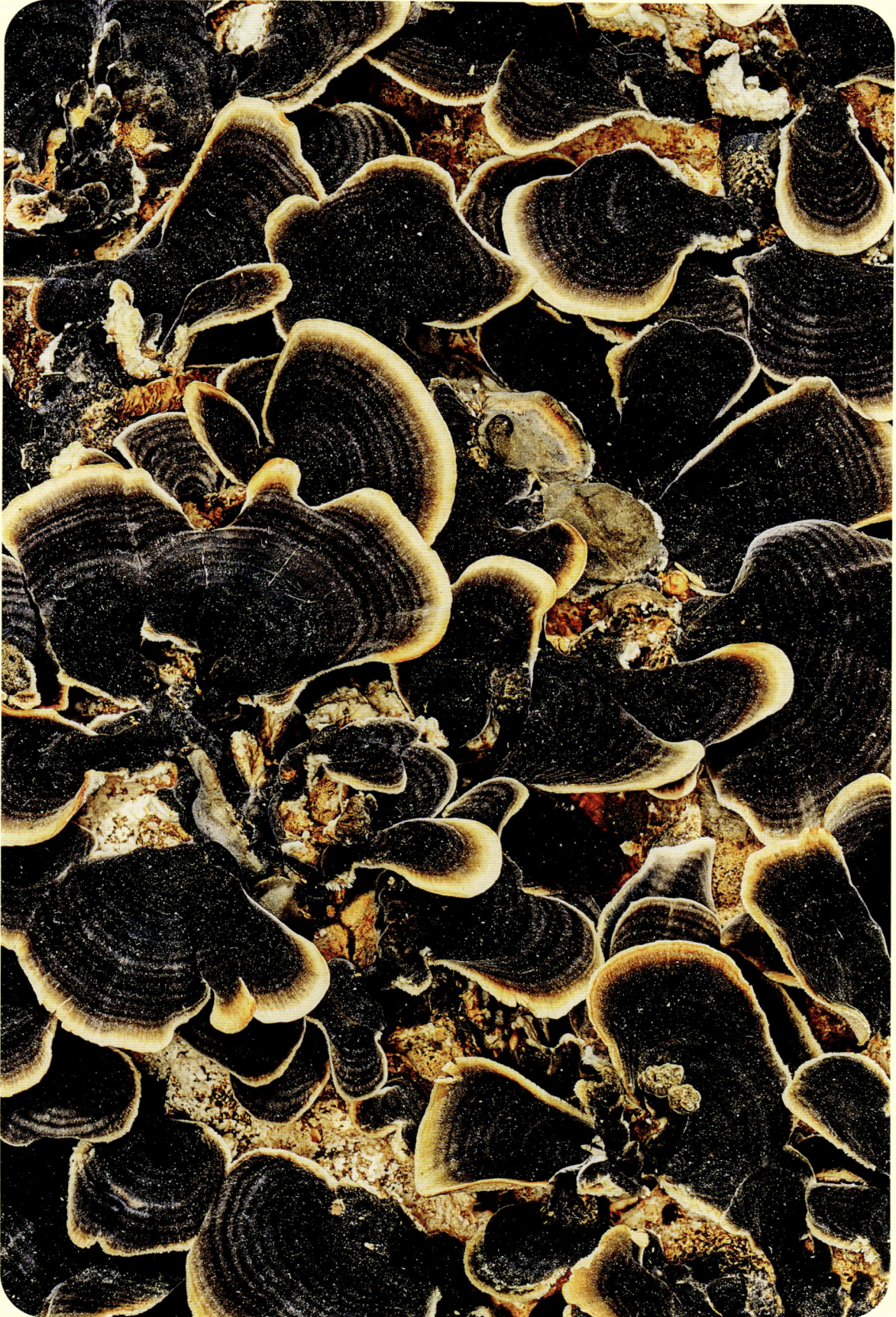

17

The Benefits and Challenges of Eating Plant-Based

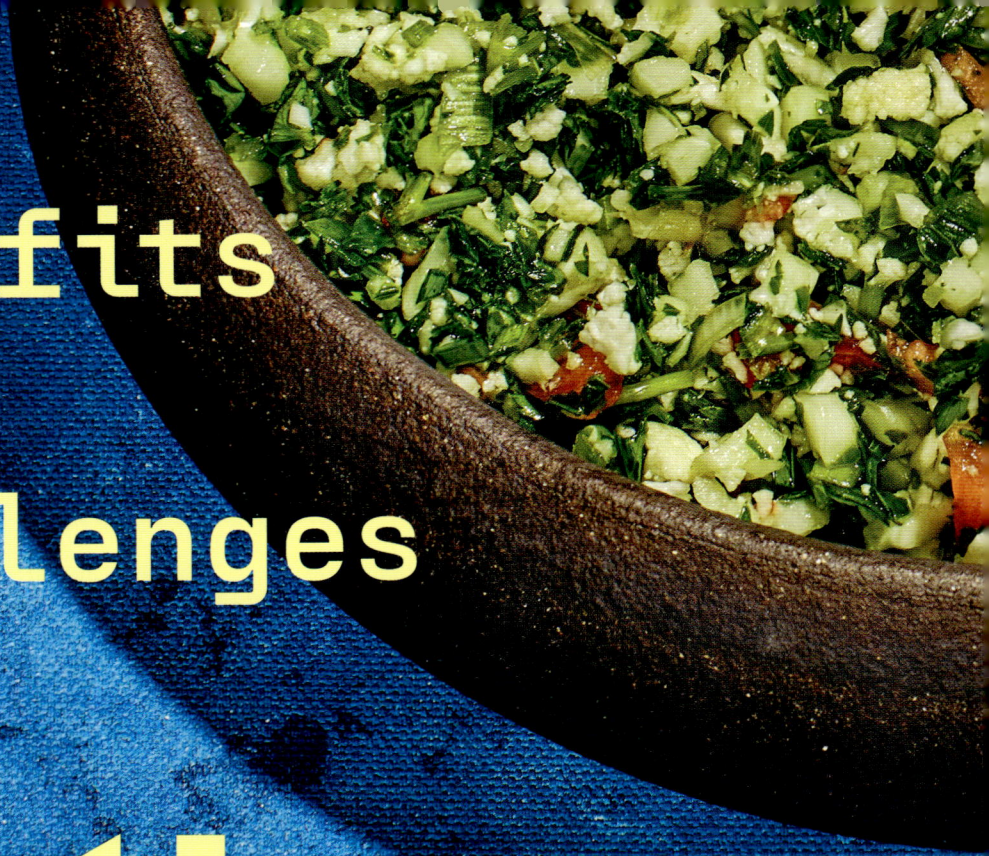

"

I started experimenting with vegetarianism at the age of twelve, and the practice of eating fewer animal products has always resonated with me. I wanted to be in the kitchen as much as possible, choosing plant-based alternatives in the grocery store, and even feeding my high school AP English class a vegetarian feast of Indian food, pasta dishes, and veggie chicken nuggets to support a paper I wrote on the subject.

In some ways, this book, more than twenty years later, feels like coming full circle. My curiosity eventually evolved and led me into the worlds of veganism and raw food, which are both exciting culinary experiences that have influenced the recipes in these pages. When I say this way of eating changed my life, I mean it literally and figuratively. Both my career and my physical health have been positively impacted. (Better digestion was a big one for me.)

While the physical benefits are profound, learning to eat with mindfulness has had positive impacts that extend beyond the plate. We live in a world where endless consumption is available, and the disconnect between food and the natural world is perpetuated by the processed food industries. While I never advocate for an all-or-nothing approach, eating plant-based (or, as I like to say, lower on the food chain) taught me how to eat seasonally and to have a deep appreciation for the natural abundance nature offers; and the biggest secret—the best-kept secret—is that these foods are better for your health.
—MEREDITH

Based on research, and personal experience, a healthy diet is all about eating diversely. When people hear "plant-based" or "healthy," they seem to think this is a limitation. However, most Americans eat only about twenty different foods in a week. This isn't a lot. When you start to eat more plant-based foods, you tend to open up your palate and start to incorporate a variety of fruits, vegetables, greens, grains, and beans, and you develop an appreciation for nature's bounty.

The Benefits

Diversity in diet matters because it automatically increases the abundance and variety of vitamins and minerals that you are consuming. If we could encourage anything, it would be to not think of this book as a call for any limitation or restriction; it is about opening a door to new and exciting ways of eating and thinking about healthier choices.

So, what are the benefits of eating plant-based? Here are just a few:

● You'll feel good in your jeans.
It's probably not surprising that a plant-based diet can help us to shed unwanted weight. Researchers have found that in multiple clinical trials, participants following a vegan diet lost an average of nine pounds and lowered their BMI by 5 to 10 percent, compared with those on control diets.[1]

● Plants are heart healthy.
Eating more plants is good for your heart too. Research participants following a vegan diet versus a control diet reduced their total cholesterol by 11.6 mg/dL, and their LDL, or "bad" cholesterol, by 9.3 mg/dL. In a separate study, participants following a vegetarian diet reduced their risk of cardiovascular disease by 15 percent, and their risk for ischemic heart disease by 21 percent, compared with non-vegetarians.[2]

● Eating plants wards off disease.
Food is our first medicine, and just by eating a diverse plant-based diet, you are taking a preventative approach to diseases like cancer and diabetes. In another series of studies, researchers found an 18 percent lower incidence of cancer in vegetarians versus non-vegetarians.[3] Data also strongly suggests a reduced risk of developing type 2 diabetes in people following vegetarian or vegan diets.[4]

● Live long and prosper.
Given the benefits listed above, it probably goes without saying that following a plant-based diet has been linked to increased longevity, not to mention improved health and quality of life during those later years. In another study of 124,706 people, researchers found a 9 percent lower risk of dying from any cause in vegetarians versus non-vegetarians.[5]

20

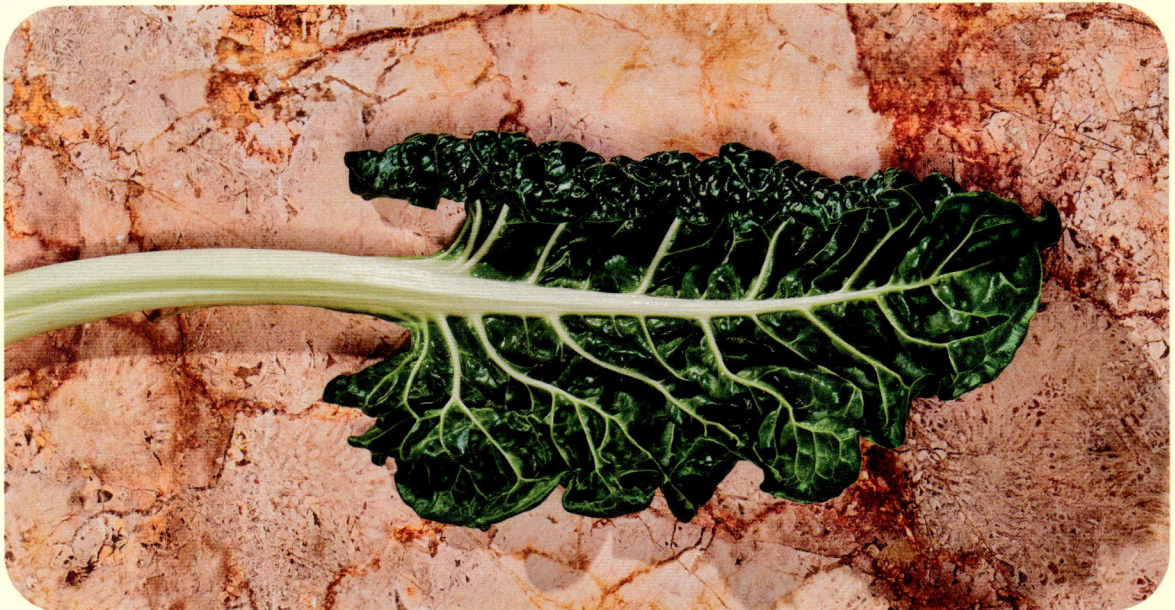

The Challenges

We are big advocates of a plant-based life and both experienced massive shifts in our overall health and energy levels when we decided to eat this way. However, we would be remiss not to address some of the challenges of following a strict plant-based diet (though we're not advocating for strict) because there are several to consider.

• Getting all your nutrients.
While it is entirely possible to meet your nutritional needs on a plant-based diet, it does require some planning and intentionality to make sure that you get all the nutrients you need in a day. If you are following a strict vegan diet, you may need to take supplements to ensure adequate intake of vitamin B12, vitamin D, and omega-3 fatty acids; B-12 is not naturally occurring in any plant-based foods, and the others are generally found in lower doses. We view quality supplementation as insurance. Being deficient in these vitamins and minerals is not limited to practicing a plant-based regimen.

• Protein quality.
Getting enough protein on a plant-based diet isn't that hard, but it is something to be mindful of. Animal sources are the most accessible forms of "complete protein," meaning that these protein sources have all nine essential amino acids. These are important building blocks for protein and protein synthesis. However, later in this chapter, we'll address how to get all nine of these essential amino acids through mixing and matching a variety of plant-based food sources, and which plant-based foods do have complete protein sources. The key to protein quality is diversity in diet and protein sources.

• Digestive issues.
Plant-based eating naturally increases your fiber intake, which is a good thing, but it can be cause for discomfort in the beginning. There is the stereotype of the "gassy vegan" for a reason. But we can promise you that with time, gradual increase in fiber intake, and improved digestion, these symptoms will go away.

• Access and availability.
It is important to acknowledge that the ease and practicality of plant-based eating is affected by where we live, our access to fresh, local produce, the general affordability of these ingredients, and the time it takes to cook. However, foods like beans and rice are affordable, healthy staples in countries around the world. When we become overly reliant on processed foods, detached from our food systems, and live in a world where vital cooking skills go unlearned, our health and well-being suffer.

• Being the only vegan at the party.
This one can be tough, especially when you are the only one at a restaurant, dinner party, or event with "dietary restrictions," and the only plant-based option on the menu is a plate of fries. Fortunately, the growing popularity and acceptance of plant-based eating is making things easier. And remember that this is not about all or nothing—if you fall off the plant-based wagon, or eating this way is not suitable for the event, don't beat yourself up.

• The plant-based learning curve.
This is something that all new plant-based eaters go through, so know that you are not alone. From mastering new cooking techniques to rethinking how to create a meal, the learning curve is real. We hope that the recipes in this book ease the transition and inspire you to think differently about how you make a plate.

Protein

The number-one question we get from people considering a plant-based diet is, *How do I make sure I get enough protein?* You may be surprised to hear that you probably don't need as much protein as you think. The recommended dietary allowance for protein is about 50 grams, equivalent to a 6-ounce chicken breast or 2 cups of lentils; most people meet this daily minimum in one meal without even trying.

Keep in mind that there are plenty of active people and even elite athletes out there whose diets are 100 percent plant based. In fact, many experts believe that following a plant-based diet improves recovery time after exercise because it helps to reduce inflammation in the body.

Different life stages (like pregnancy) or levels of activity may call for more focused and elevated protein requirements. If you are a full-time plant-based eater and concerned about protein intake, consider methods to increase protein, such as high-quality protein powders, including soy products; sprinkling salads with high-protein sources like hemp seeds; and consciously adding a high-quality source to each meal to ensure an adequate amino acid profile in your diet. This essentially means increasing the diversity of your protein sources to maximize the quality and variety.

What is a complete protein?

We hear that plant-based proteins are "incomplete" because they do not contain adequate levels of all nine essential amino acids necessary in the human diet. However, it's easy to get all of your amino acids in a plant-based diet simply by mixing and matching a variety of plant-based protein sources throughout the day. Soy is the exception and is often considered a plant-based hero ingredient, because it contains all nine essential amino acids that the body cannot produce on its own. This makes it one of the best plant-based protein sources, comparable to animal proteins in terms of amino acid profile.

The list opposite shows you the nine essential amino acids and the foods that most commonly contain them. This information can feel intimidating, or like it requires a lot of calculation, but, as with everything when it comes to healthy eating, focusing on diversity and quality of ingredients will help you meet your needs.

Essential amino acids can be categorized based on their chemical properties, and one of these properties is sulfur content. Among the nine essential amino acids, only one contains sulfur. This distinction isn't something you need to spend a lot of time thinking about, but it matters because they do play different roles in the body, especially when it comes to protein. The simplest breakdown is that sulfur-containing amino acids are critical for protein stability and regulation, while the non-sulfur amino acids are more generalized in maintaining the protein structure.

> **NON-SULFUR-CONTAINING ESSENTIAL AMINO ACIDS**

This list is limited to the essential amino acids.

→ **HISTIDINE**
meat, poultry, fish, dairy, and some grains

→ **ISOLEUCINE**
meat, poultry, fish, eggs, dairy, soy products, legumes, nuts, and seeds

→ **LEUCINE**
meat, poultry, fish, dairy, soy products, legumes, nuts, and seeds

→ **LYSINE**
meat, poultry, fish, dairy, soy products, legumes, quinoa, and pumpkin seeds

→ **PHENYLALANINE**
meat, poultry, fish, eggs, dairy, soy products, legumes, nuts, and seeds

→ **THREONINE**
meat, poultry, fish, dairy, soy products, legumes, nuts, and seeds

→ **TRYPTOPHAN**
meat, poultry, fish, dairy, eggs, soy products, legumes, nuts, and seeds

→ **VALINE**
meat, poultry, fish, dairy, soy products, legumes, nuts, and seeds

SULFUR-CONTAINING ESSENTIAL AMINO ACID

→ **METHIONINE**
meat, poultry, fish, eggs, dairy, soy products, legumes, nuts, and seeds

* A note about methionine:
Methionine is the primary sulfur-containing essential amino acid, the primary non-essential being cysteine. Sulfur-containing amino acids are essential for protein synthesis.

* A note about lysine:
Lysine is the one amino acid that is hardest to get on a plant-based diet. While many plant-based foods contain lysine, they are typically in lower amounts than those found in animal products. Therefore, it is important to consume a daily variety of plant foods known to have higher lysine content, such as legumes (beans, lentils, peas), quinoa, pumpkin seeds, and soy-based products like tofu and tempeh. Combining these foods with grains to get a balance of the other, sulfur-containing amino acids, such as methionine and cysteine, is important because these amino acids work together to support various critical functions in the body like protein synthesis, collagen production, immune system support, and metabolic function.

23

AMINO ACID CHART

% RDA PER 100 GRAMS	BEEF SIRLOIN	WHITE BEANS	SOYBEANS	COOKED PEAS	RICE
Histidine	128%	29%	64%	15%	9%
Isoleucine	91%	23%	58%	14%	8%
Leucine	82%	21%	50%	12%	8%
Lysine	113%	24%	53%	15%	5%
Methionine	113%	16%	32%	12%	9%
Phenylalanine	48%	17%	38%	9%	5%
Threonine	107%	29%	69%	19%	9%
Tryptophan	66%	31%	86%	13%	11%
Valine	76%	21%	46%	13%	9%

Below is a list of plant-based proteins and the essential amino acids that they include.[6] If your daily plant-based meals include items from the categories below, you won't have any trouble getting all nine of the essentials.

1. Grains and cereals like rice are typically deficient in lysine but contain high levels of the sulfur-containing amino acids cysteine and methionine. Here are some of our favorite grains that contain the most complete essential amino acid profiles—some include lysine:

- **AMARANTH**
Complete protein that contains lysine.

- **QUINOA**
Often considered a complete protein, quinoa has a higher lysine content compared to most other grains.

- **TEFF**
An ancient grain from Ethiopia that also has a higher lysine content compared to more commonly consumed grains; it's great to use in baking.

2. Vegetables and legumes (including beans, peanuts, chickpeas, etc.) are generally lower in sulfur-containing amino acids like cysteine and methionine but richer in lysine. Some examples of high-lysine vegetables and legumes are:

- **AVOCADO** (though technically a fruit)
- **BROCCOLI**
- **KALE**
- **SPINACH**

3. Nuts and seeds are usually low in lysine but contain many other essential amino acids, with the exception of pumpkin seeds, which are relatively high in lysine.

4. Soy protein is regarded as the most complete vegan amino acid source. It contains all nine essential amino acids in sufficient quantities to meet our dietary needs, making it a high-quality plant-based protein option. Soy protein is versatile and can be incorporated into a variety of products such as tofu, tempeh, and soy milk. And of course, it's in everyone's favorite snack, edamame.

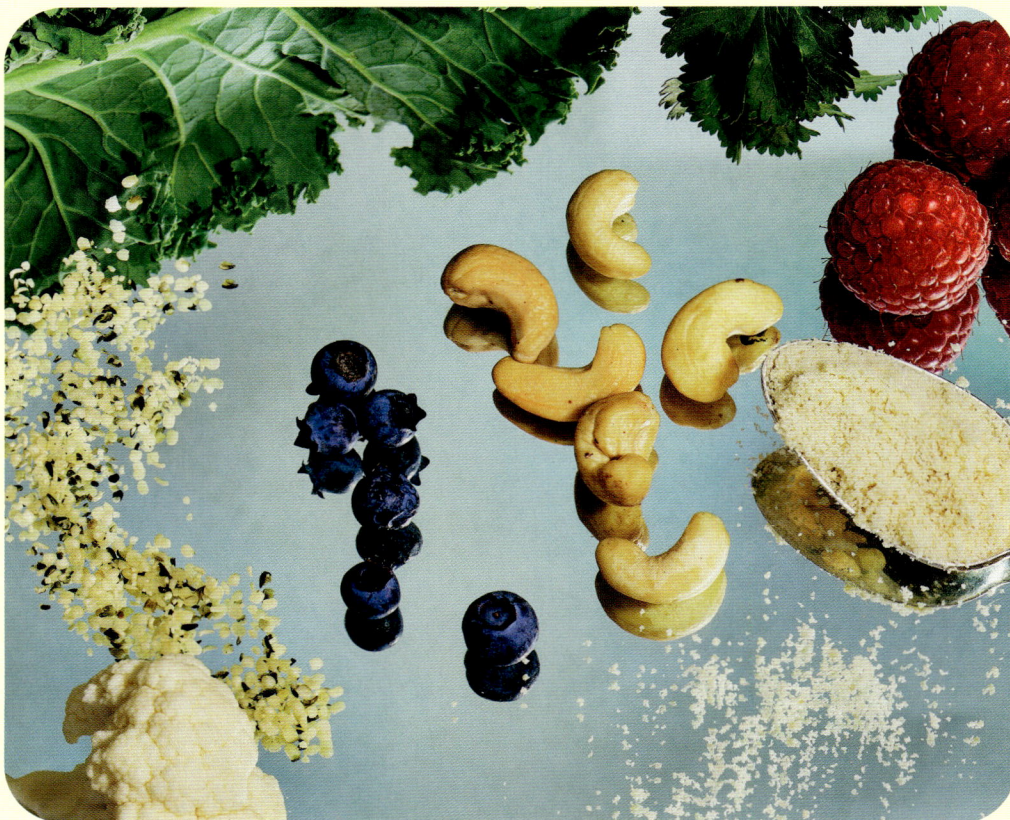

Blueprint for a
Balanced Smoothie

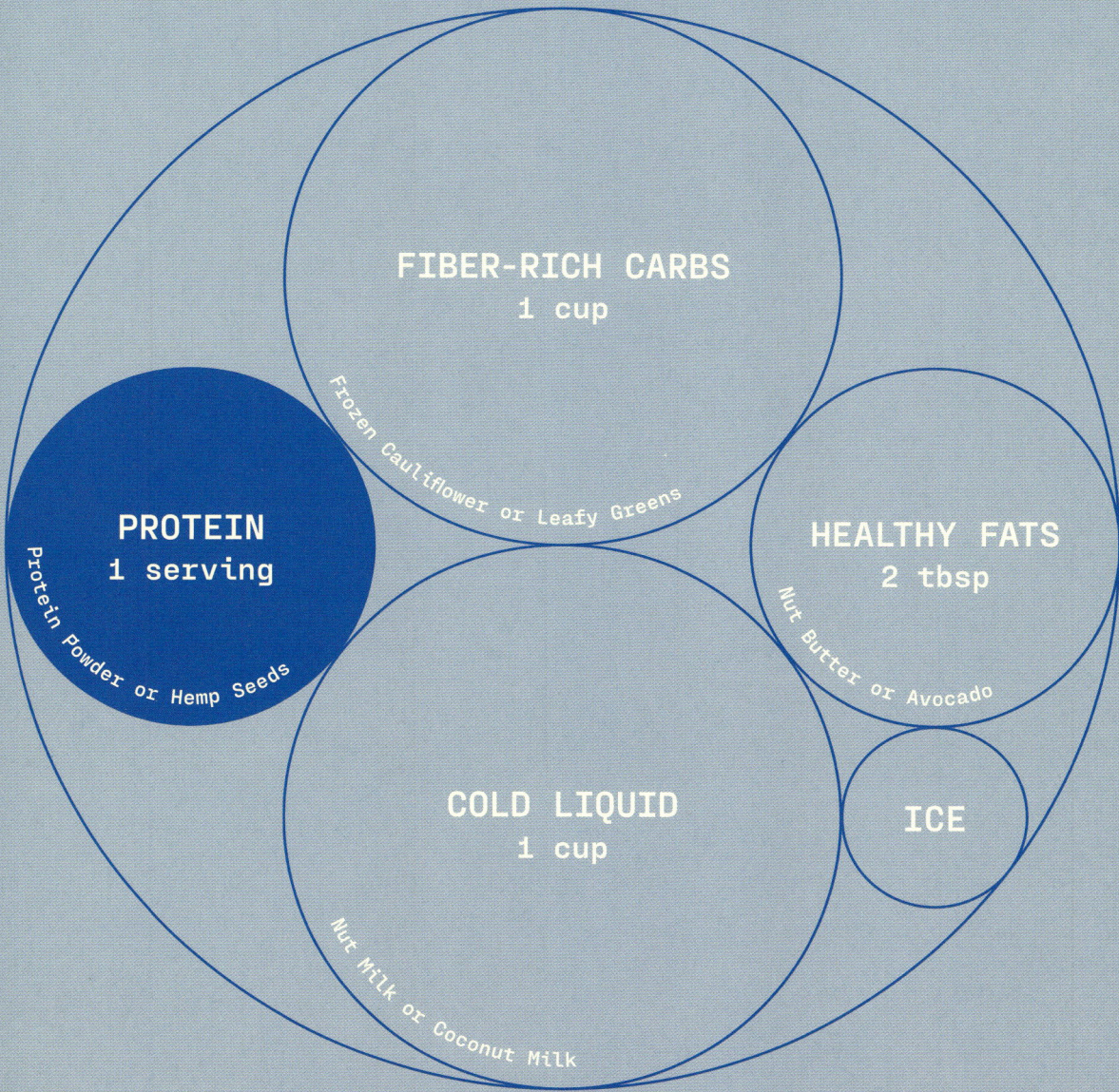

FIBER-RICH CARBS
1 cup

Frozen Cauliflower or Leafy Greens

HEALTHY FATS
2 tbsp

Nut Butter or Avocado

PROTEIN
1 serving

Protein Powder or Hemp Seeds

COLD LIQUID
1 cup

Nut Milk or Coconut Milk

ICE

PANTRY

Now for the fun part—
it's time to stock your pantry and fridge!

With the ingredients listed on
hand, you'll be ready to make a variety
of healthy, delicious, plant-based meals
in a matter of minutes.

STAPLES

● PLANT-BASED
PANTRY STAPLES

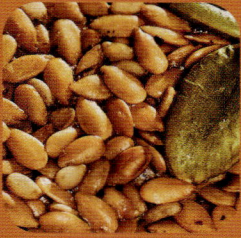

WHOLE GRAINS

NUT & SEED BUTTERS

HERBS & SPICES

COCONUT MILK

HEALTHY OILS

WHOLE GRAIN PASTAS, BROWN RICE,
GLASS NOODLES & RICE PAPER

SEAWEED

CANNED TOMATOES & TOMATO PASTE

BEANS—DRIED & CANNED

NUTS & SEEDS

27

● FRIDGE STAPLES

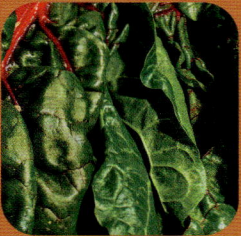

LETTUCES & GREENS

HERBS

FRESH VEGETABLES

FRESH FRUIT

TOFU & TEMPEH

MISO PASTE

DIJON MUSTARD

NAMA SHOYU OR TAMARI

OLIVES

KRAUT & KIMCHI

Plant-Based Pantry Staples

WHOLE GRAINS

Whole grains like whole wheat, quinoa, oats, brown rice, amaranth, and teff are a great source of dietary fiber that offer many health benefits, such as regulating digestion and blood sugar, and benefiting your cardio health. We'll get into this more in Chapter 2: Help Your Self Love Your Gut.

According to research, however, 97 percent of men and 94 percent of women are not meeting the daily recommendations for dietary fiber intake (roughly 25 g for adult women and 28 g for adult men), even though these numbers are relatively low.

We would recommend eating more than the DV. Whole grains are a great source of fiber, whereas refined grains (like white rice and white flour) are less so because of the significant processing they undergo.

NUT AND SEED BUTTERS

Slathered on fruit, toast, crackers, and more, the nut butter options are endless. But our favorite way to use them is in dressings and sauces. See our recipe for Better Nut Butter Sauce (page 45). We put it on everything.

HERBS AND SPICES

We generally find that less is more when it comes to spices. Have a spice cabinet full of dried spices that are well past their prime? Just let them go. Clean it up and clean it out. Then invest in a few high-quality spices that can't be replaced by fresh herbs. We always have chili powder, turmeric powder, cumin, coriander, oregano, thyme, cinnamon, cardamom, and a good curry powder on hand. Most leafy herbs lose their flavor when dried, so dried herbs like parsley, basil, and mint are a waste of money and space in our opinion. Stock your spice cabinet with some good sea salt and pepper too.

COCONUT MILK

This stuff has so many uses and can be added to coffee, soups, dressings, curries, and more for a hint of delicious coconut-y creaminess. Make sure to look for the unsweetened varieties with no guar added.

HEALTHY OILS

These include organic olive oil, avocado oil, sesame oil, walnut oil, pumpkin seed oil, hemp seed oil, coconut oil, and others. When choosing an oil, it is most important to consider the quality and to opt for cold-pressed organic varieties. For cooking or finishing a salad, it's great to have a variety on hand. Experiment to find your favorites.

WHOLE GRAIN PASTAS, BROWN RICE, GLASS NOODLES, AND RICE PAPER

These are all healthy dried goods that can be added in the rotation, and it is nice to mix up your grain sources. As much as we love rice, we all know that noodles hit differently with their versatility and universal appeal.

SEAWEED

Dried seaweed is essential to have on hand, as a snack, for making broths, for sprinkling on salads, and for making quick sandwich wraps.

CANNED TOMATOES AND TOMATO PASTE

Canned tomatoes are one of those ingredients that can easily transform any meal. And a flavorful dollop of tomato paste changes everything when you add it to beans or rice. See our delicious recipe for Lentil and Tempeh Bolognese (page 144).

BEANS—DRIED AND CANNED

Cooking beans is not hard, but not being gassy after eating them can be. That's why we recommend buying dried beans and then soaking and pressure cooking them to remove lectins and antinutrients, which are partly to blame for making them hard to digest.

These "antinutrients," such as phytic acid and lectins, can interfere with the absorption of certain nutrients but are reduced through soaking, cooking, or fermentation. In the wild, these compounds serve as natural protection so that the seeds can germinate and grow under optimal conditions, but on the plate, they can make the beans harder to digest. With proper preparation, they are easy to eliminate in the cooking process.

We won't blame you for relying on good ol' canned beans sometimes, but remember that they may contain a higher sodium content, and always look for BPA-free cans. If you need to go canned, look for organic and low-salt varieties that you can have on hand as healthy pantry staples in a pinch.

NUTS AND SEEDS

Many of the recipes in this book offer unique ways to use nuts and seeds, including making your own nut milks and meat alternatives. There are also lots of other simple ways to add healthy nuts and seeds to your diet that require no recipe at all. Have some hemp seeds in the pantry? Sprinkle them on a salad. Steamed kale? Add chopped walnuts. You're already on your way to a healthier meal.

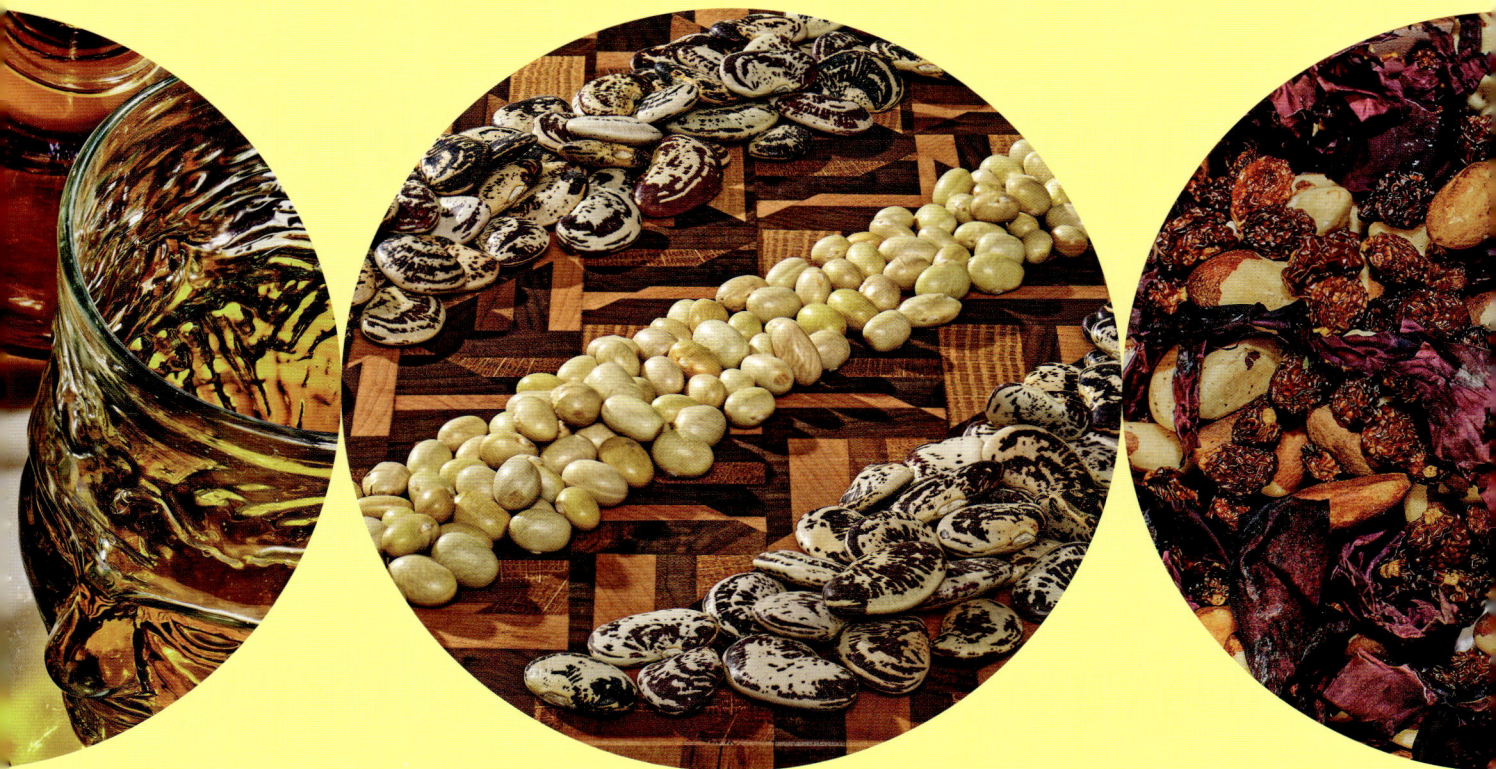

29

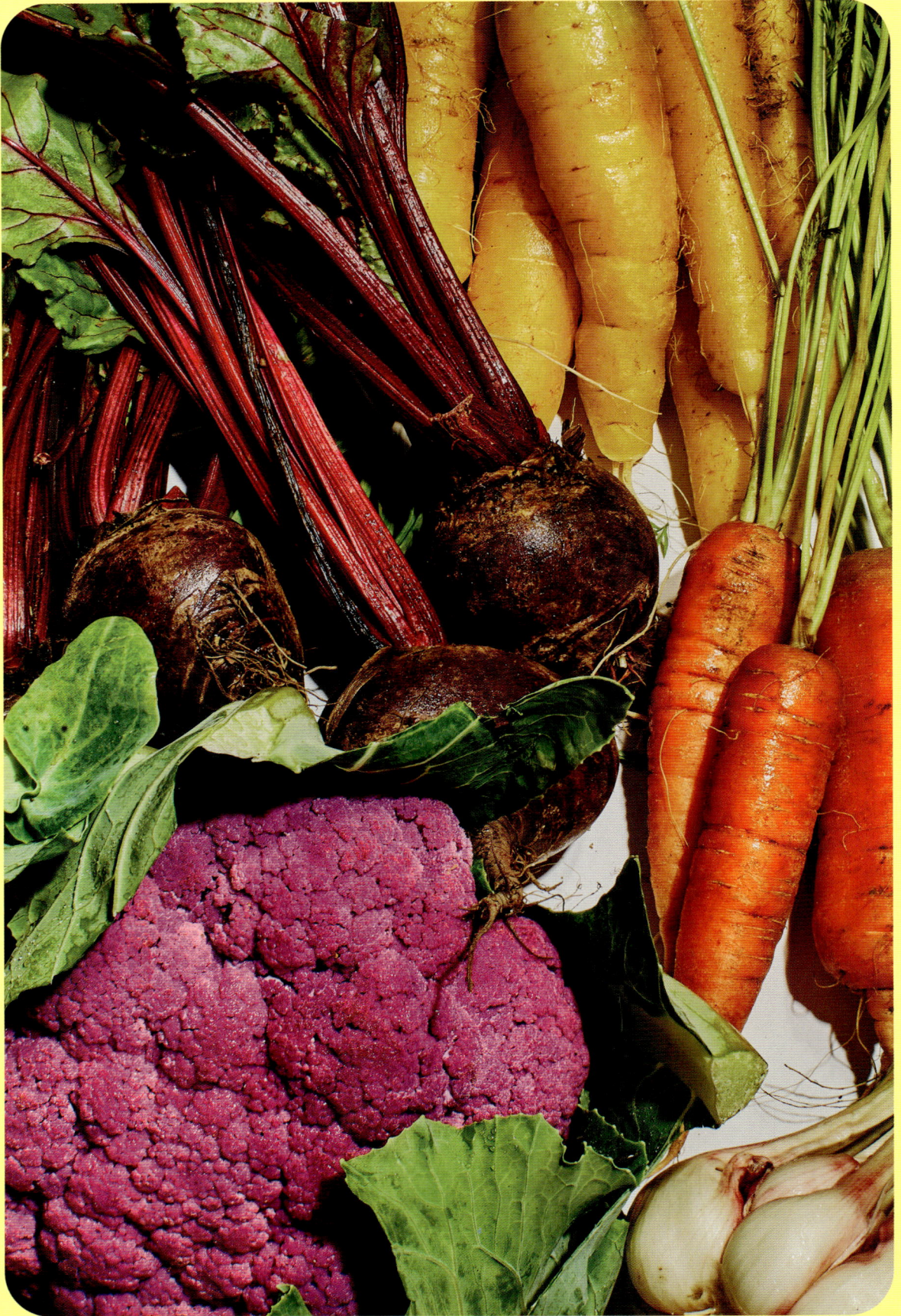

30

Fridge Staples

LETTUCES AND GREENS

Reframing a meal around lettuces and greens is not some fad diet move. Greens are hydrating, high in fiber, and rich in flavor, and they come in so many exquisite varieties and taste delicious. Be adventurous, and remember, your greens don't have to be green! We love all the purple, pink, burgundy, and bronze lettuces you can find in the fall. Eating a variety of colors in your diet is a great way to ensure diversity in vitamin and mineral content.

HERBS

Packed with flavor and medicinal benefits, fresh, chopped herbs can be game changing for any dish. Sprinkle on some chopped basil, scallions, chives, mint—you name it. And you don't have to follow a recipe to use them on the regular. The more the merrier when it comes to fresh herbs.

FRESH VEGETABLES

Of course, we must include fresh veggies. Our favorites to keep on hand that serve a variety of functions are cauliflower, broccoli, zucchini, and carrots.

MUSHROOMS

Although they are most often classified as vegetables, mushrooms technically occupy their own category—the fungus. As one of our favorite meaty alternatives, mushrooms have a wide array of health benefits and culinary uses. We encourage you to get experimental and try new varieties when you have the chance.

FRESH FRUIT

Fruit is your friend. Fresh fruit is one of the most nutritious foods on the planet. We recommend eating it alone, or before a meal instead of at the end for the best digestion.

TOFU AND TEMPEH

The addition of a little tofu and tempeh can really help boost the satisfaction of a meal. It doesn't take much. All you have to do is grill a few slices with olive oil and a pinch of sea salt, and then add them to bowls or salads, put them in a tortilla, or just dip them in sauce and enjoy.

MISO PASTE

Miso makes a great addition to so many dishes, giving them that delicious umami boost. Because it's fermented, it also lasts forever in the fridge, so we recommend stocking a variety of types, from chickpea miso for a light and versatile soy-free version, to darker, more aged miso for depth of flavor. And miso isn't just for Asian-style dishes—there are so many uses for it. Try adding a tablespoon to blended soups, dressings, pasta sauces, you name it . . . anywhere you need a little salty depth of flavor.

DIJON MUSTARD

Meredith once claimed that mustard was her favorite food, and while she has since revised this statement, it is still one of the most versatile refrigerator condiments to add a hit of flavor to almost anything.

NAMA SHOYU OR TAMARI

For a splash of mineral-rich flavor, we love nama shoyu, which is raw and unpasteurized soy sauce. Keep in mind that it does contain wheat. Tamari is a similar option that is generally wheat-free. There are gluten-free soy sauces that make good options as well. While there are subtle flavor differences, you'll win a prize if you can tell.

OLIVES

Versatile, flavorful, and full of healthy fats, the olive can't be overrated. If you haven't tried cured Botija olives, they might just change your life.

KRAUT AND KIMCHI

For a salty hit of fermented flavor that also has huge benefits for your gut health, try adding a small side of sauerkraut or kimchi to a dish. Eating these items is more traditional in other cultures, but we've fully adopted them and eat one or the other with almost every meal.

Rethinking the Food Pyramid

We all remember learning about the food pyramid in school, with a giant pile of bread, rice, and pasta at its base. The food pyramid was created in the 1970s with the intention of helping people to make informed choices about their nutrition, and it is sorely in need of an update. What many of us don't realize is that the pyramid is heavily influenced by food industry lobbies, and the recommendations are often skewed based on the support of these industries.[7] Our understanding of nutrition has evolved, and the food pyramid has some catching-up to do.

We're not fans of the traditional food pyramid for the following reasons:

- It lacks nuance and relies too heavily on food category generalizations.

- It overemphasizes animal products and has limited recognition of plant-based protein.

- It fails to differentiate between whole and refined grains.

- It fails to differentiate between whole and refined grains.

- It shows an inadequate representation of healthy fats (from avocados, nuts, seeds, and olives)—all fats are listed together as "use sparingly."

As we've stated, we are in desperate need of an updated dietary framework that addresses the issues listed above and includes more nuance and variety in its recommendations.

As we see it, this updated framework should include:

- A VARIETY OF PLANT-BASED OPTIONS.
An updated dietary model should emphasize inclusivity and variety by promoting a wide range of fresh and seasonal plant-based foods.

- PLANT-BASED PROTEIN REQUIREMENTS.
Acknowledging the viability of plant-based protein sources is imperative to a modern and updated approach to nutrition, particularly in a world where we are dealing with chronic health issues, questions of sustainability, and climate change.

- THE DISTINGUISHING OF HEALTHY FATS.
Recognizing the difference between healthy and unhealthy fats is essential. By encouraging the consumption of whole-food plant-based sources like avocados, nuts, and olive oil, we acknowledge the nuance.

- ENVIRONMENTAL CONSIDERATIONS.
Our new plant-based pyramid considers the environmental impact of our food choices. According to the United Nations Food and Agriculture Organization (FAO), a plant-based diet may reduce greenhouse gas emissions significantly, as livestock production accounts for approximately 14.5 percent of global emissions, more than all transportation combined. Additionally, a global shift to a plant-based diet could free up to 75 percent of agricultural land, allowing for reforestation and biodiversity restoration.

32

The New Plant-Based Food Pyramid

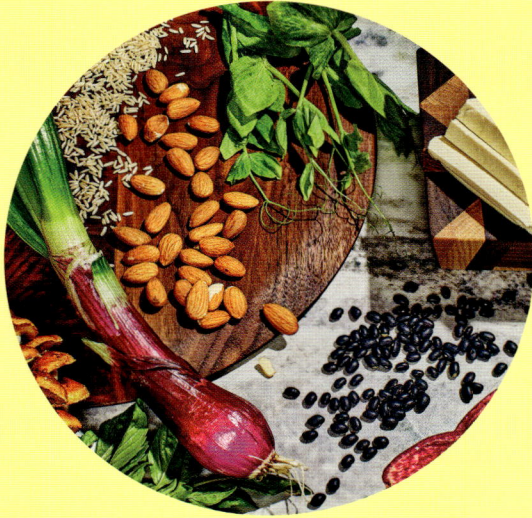

This pyramid should serve as a daily guide. If you pull from each of these categories at every meal, you will be in a great place. Physical activity and hydration should make up the foundation of any healthy routine, because they are fundamental to good health.

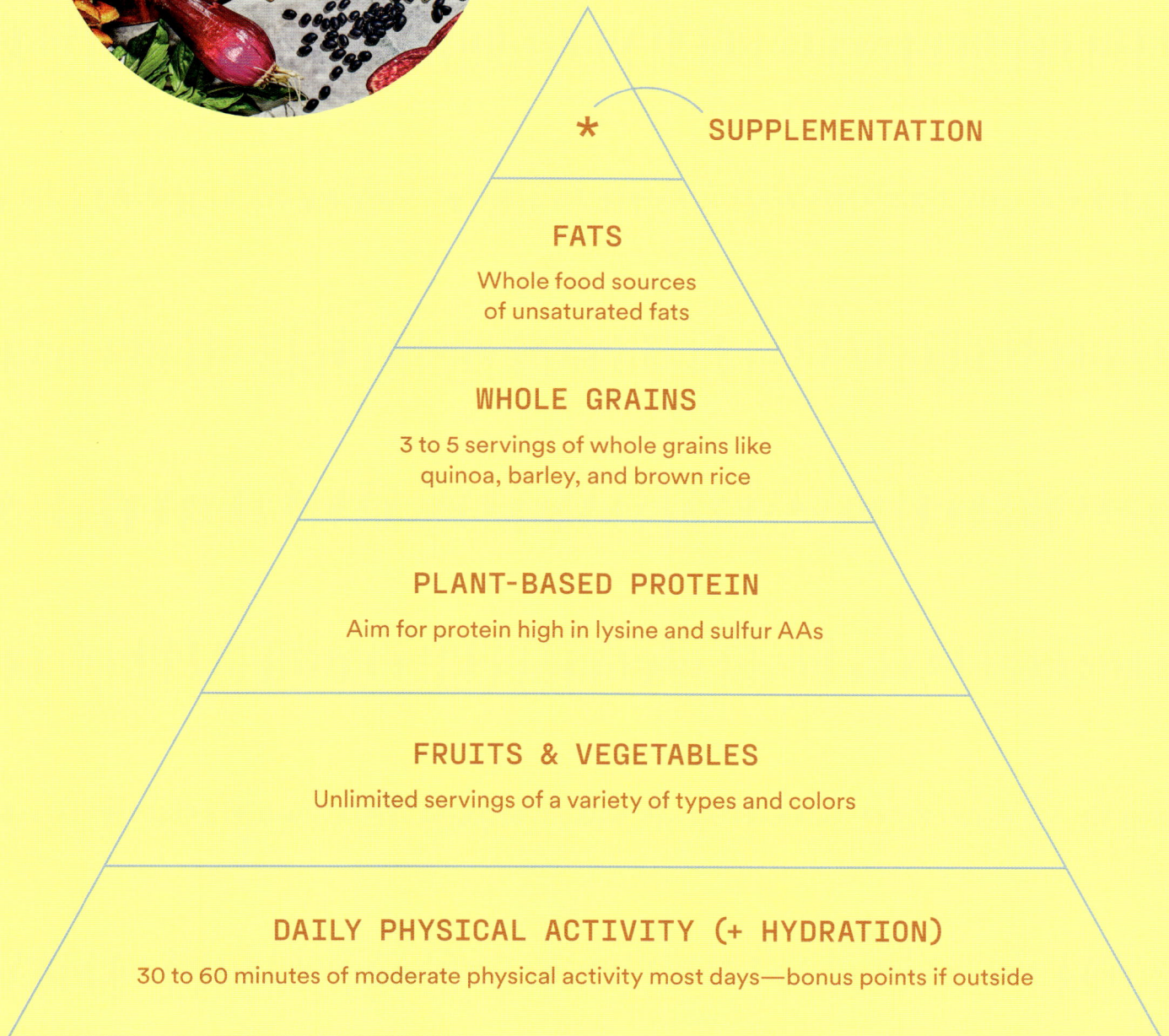

*   **SUPPLEMENTATION**

FATS

Whole food sources
of unsaturated fats

WHOLE GRAINS

3 to 5 servings of whole grains like
quinoa, barley, and brown rice

PLANT-BASED PROTEIN

Aim for protein high in lysine and sulfur AAs

FRUITS & VEGETABLES

Unlimited servings of a variety of types and colors

DAILY PHYSICAL ACTIVITY (+ HYDRATION)

30 to 60 minutes of moderate physical activity most days—bonus points if outside

Did You Say Soy?

We know there's been some controversy over soy. One day it was in as a health food staple, and then the next day it was out. But we never stopped eating it. Many of the healthiest cultures in the world have long consumed soy as part of a balanced diet, regardless of food trends, and the research backs up its health benefits.

Some people have concerns that soy has a negative impact on hormonal health, as it contains phytoestrogens, plant-based substances that mimic estrogen and can alter hormone levels. But overall, the data does not show negative effects of soy consumption on hormone levels or function in men or women. A 2021 meta-analysis of forty-one clinical trials, conducted mostly in Western populations, found that soy had no effect on reproductive hormone levels in men.[8]

For women, the very point of concern may in fact be a beneficial aspect, as research reveals that such benefits as enhanced bone health, relief from menopausal hot flashes, and improved cognitive function may stem from consuming soy.[9] (Some of these benefits apply to men as well.) The scientific data also indicates that soy has either no impact, or a protective influence, on cardiovascular events and breast cancer. Please note that these benefits lie in the organic and non-GMO soy versions, not in the soy that is used in processed-food production. Good news, soy consumers!

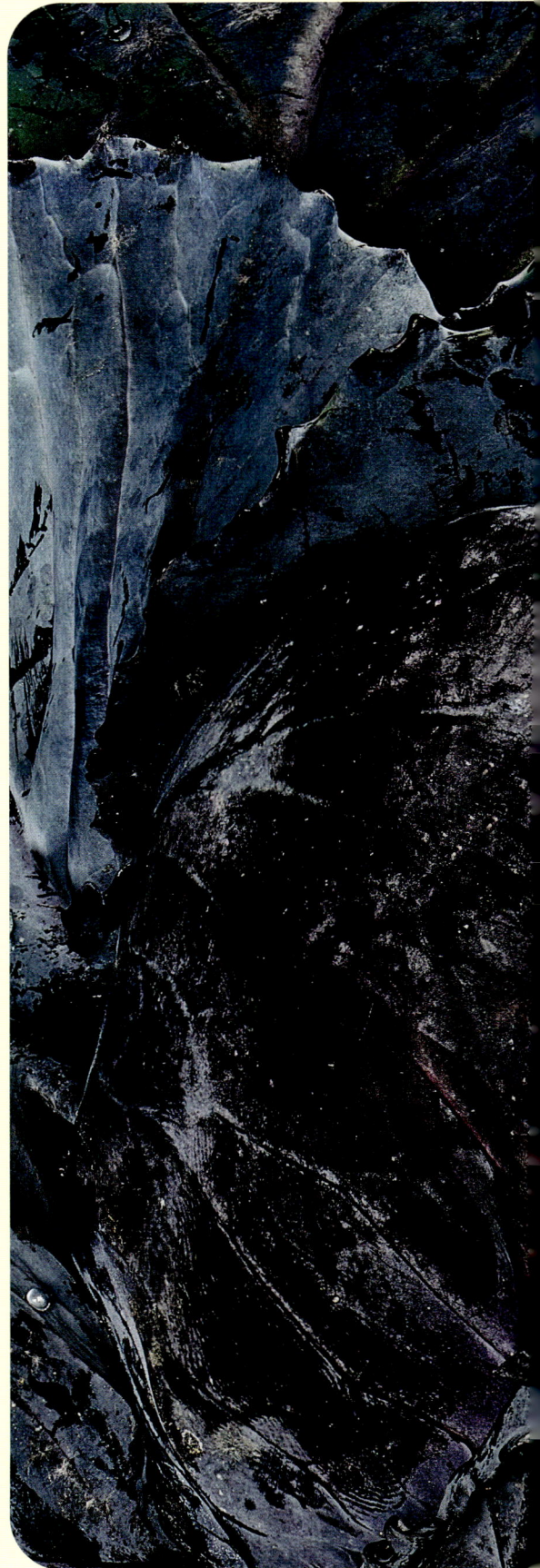

35

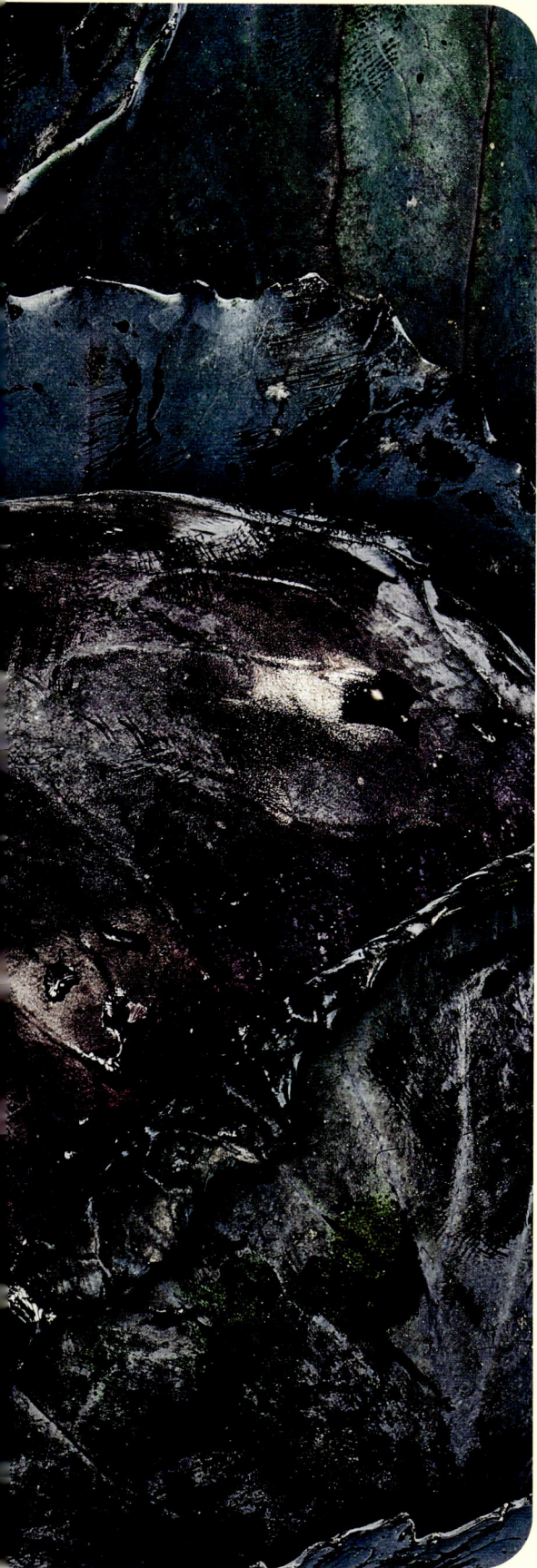

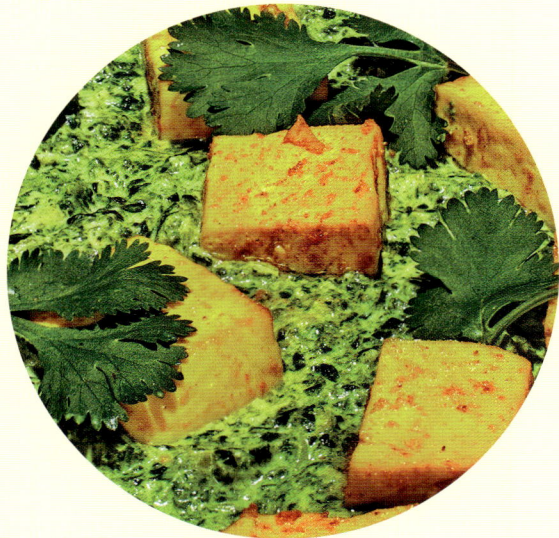

What about GMOs?

The other point of contention around soy consumption is the notion that it is a primarily GMO (or genetically modified) food. In truth, it's quite easy to find organic, GMO-free soy products in high-quality tofu, tempeh, fermented soy sauces, and soy milks. The issue of GMO soy comes into play when soy is used as an additive in processed foods, and in animal feed.

There is an irony in avoiding soy products because of GMOs while still eating an animal foods–based diet because roughly 70 to 80 percent of GMO soybeans grown in the United States are used for animal feed. Nonorganic cow's milk, cheese, and meat are all vessels for GMO soy consumption and are most likely the only reason to be concerned about soy. Again, the emphasis on whole organic soy foods—very different from getting it secondhand in food production.

Seed Oils

If you pay any attention to health trends, you've probably heard that "seed oils" are the latest villains. Seed oils are refined vegetable oils that come from the seeds of plants, and they are extracted by pressing. They are popular for cooking, especially at high temperatures, because of their neutral taste and high smoke point.

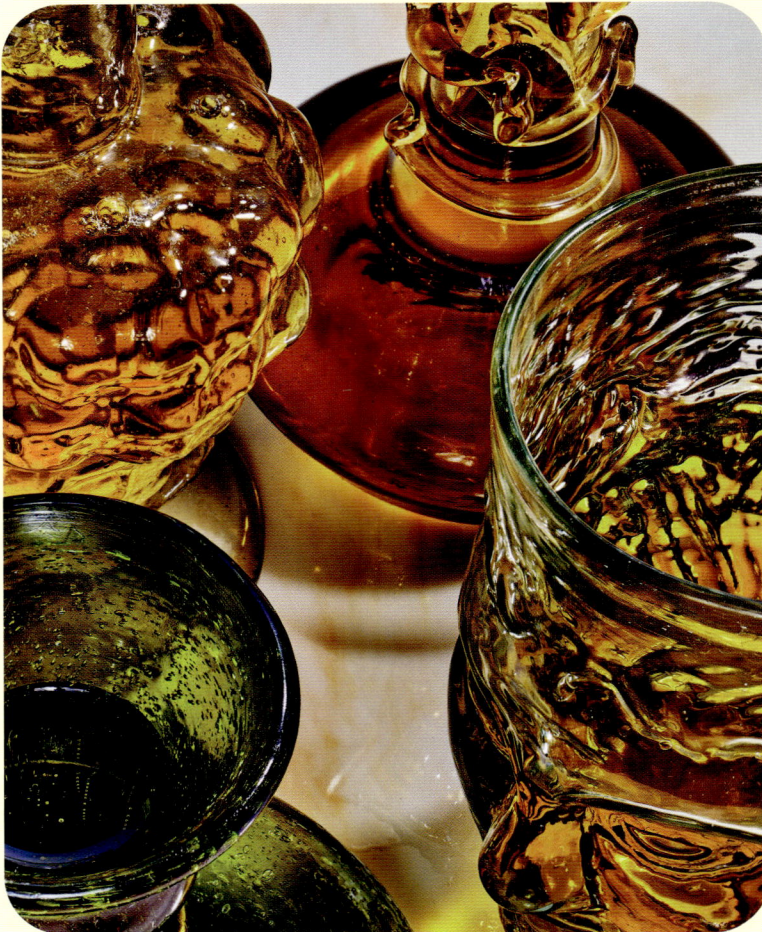

They include:

→ CANOLA OIL

→ CORN OIL

→ COTTONSEED OIL

→ GRAPESEED OIL

→ PEANUT OIL

→ RICE-BRAN OIL

→ SAFFLOWER OIL

→ SOYBEAN OIL

→ SUNFLOWER OIL

* OLIVE, AVOCADO, AND COCONUT OILS COME FROM THE FRUIT OF THE SOURCE AND ARE THERE-FORE NOT CONSIDERED SEED OILS.

The Fatty Acid Debate

One of the health concerns surrounding seed oils stems from many of them having a high ratio of omega-6 to omega-3 fatty acids, more than 50:1 in many cases. Omega-6 fatty acid is an essential fatty acid that our bodies need and that we cannot synthesize, so we have to get it from our diet. The trouble is that whereas traditional diets (before the introduction of highly processed foods) have a ratio of 1:1 of omega-3s to omega-6s, modern diets, which include lots of seed oil–containing processed foods, are more like 15:1.[10] It is possible that an imbalance of omega-6s to omega-3s, linked to seed oils, may increase inflammation.

Processing

The next concern over seed oils—and we see this as a big one—has to do with how they are processed. A cold-pressed oil is always going to have more integrity, and be better quality, than a highly processed and ultra-refined oil. These processing methods are not limited to seed oil extraction, but commercially processed seed oils are the ones that are most commonly compromised. Common extraction methods used in commercial seed oil production include centrifuging (spinning at high speed), crushing or pressing (typical for flax or hemp seed oil), and chemical extraction (using solvents). Solvent extraction with hexane is the standard practice in today's modern processing facilities for most commercially used seed oils and is the one extraction method to try to avoid. The 1990 Clean Air Act listed hexane as a hazardous air pollutant, but manufacturers resist change because of efficiency advantages of hexane over less toxic options.[11] Do you want that in your food? We don't.

So how do you avoid seed oils extracted by solvents?

• Look for organic. Organic oils are typically processed without hexane.

• Avoid or minimize processed foods.

• Read labels and look for "cold-pressed" or "expeller-pressed."

Heat

Seed oils are often referred to as "RBD oils," which refers to the process by which they are manufactured: refined, bleached, deodorized (RBD). Refining is a multistep process involving removal of phospholipids (degumming), removal of free fatty acids (deacidification), removal of pigments, removal of other impurities (decolorization), and removal of odors (deodorization). This process involves high heat, which can increase trans-fatty acid content and reduce beneficial components like antioxidants and plant sterols.[12] The end result is a far cry from what nature intended.

For refined seed oils, heat is not only a factor in the extraction method; it is of course also used in cooking and frying at high temperatures. Repeated heating of seed oils, as is done with restaurant deep fryers, results in harmful compounds that occur when fat is oxidized during heating.[13] This is not specific to seed oils, but since they are most used for frying, the problem is more focused on them.

All you need to know is that choosing cold-pressed or expeller-pressed oils is the best way to avoid oils that have been extracted using solvents or heated. Processed foods are most often the real culprit here. If a food contains an organic and cold-pressed seed oil—like grapeseed, sunflower seed, sesame seed, flax or hemp seed—we believe it can be included as part of a healthy and balanced diet, because it still retains integrity as a whole food.

Allergen Concerns

It is important to note that most industrial seed oils are labeled as "vegetable oil," and common sources of vegetable oil include soybeans, corn, canola, sunflower seeds, safflower seeds, cotton seeds, peanuts, and olives. If you have any of these allergens, it is very hard to avoid cross-contamination when eating in restaurants or consuming processed foods that contain vegetable oil.

What's the Takeaway on Seed Oils?

Our take on this debate is that while individual seed oils can be part of a balanced diet, it's essential to consume them in moderation, with your focus on the minimally processed versions, and on a wide variety without being overly reliant on just one type of oil. Eating fried food in restaurants is a common source of "bad" oils, and while we would never tell anyone to give up French fries for life, it is worth acknowledging that these types of fried foods are a consistent source of refined seed oil exposure.

How Clean Is Your Cookware?

Like food trends, cookware trends come and go. When it comes to cookware, we tend to apply much of the same wisdom that we would for trendy food rules. We like to take a step back and look at what has traditionally and consistently been used over time—in the case of cookware, this means natural materials that are tried and true. Glass, stainless-steel, cast-iron, wooden, and some ceramic materials are the varieties of cookware that win in our homes.

Using safe cookware is an important consideration for maintaining both your health and the integrity of your food. The good news is that natural materials are relatively easy to find, and they are often less expensive than some of the newer materials.

What makes a material unsafe for cooking? Leaching, reactivity, toxicity, flammability, and tendency to corrode are all factors that play into determining whether cookware is safe to use, aka "clean."

CLEAN COOKWARE WE LOVE

When it comes to nontoxic cookware, the options can be overwhelming. And while we'd like to say that focusing on natural materials is the way forward, it is a little more complicated than that. Getting into the weeds on trendy materials can be a waste of time. Instead, we'd like to recommend simplifying by focusing on the classics: stainless steel, cast iron, and glass.

Stainless steel

As far as we are concerned, stainless steel is the gold standard for clean cookware. Durable, corrosion resistant, and nonreactive, stainless steel hits all the marks. It is slightly harder to cook with, and decidedly not nonstick, but once you get the hang of using it, there is no problem.

Cast iron

Known for its durability, everlasting quality, and ability to retain heat, cast iron is a constant go-to for us. When properly seasoned, a natural nonstick surface forms on cast iron, which makes it ideal for cooking most dishes without a chemical coating. We prefer not to cook with acid in the cast-iron, as it can be reactive to acidic ingredients like tomato sauce or lots of lemon.

Enameled cast iron

All the benefits of cast iron with a porcelain enamel coating that functions as a nonstick-like surface (although not entirely nonstick) without chemicals. The con of enameled cast iron is that it is heavy and often a feature of premium brands like Le Creuset and Staub.

Glass

Glass cookware is entirely inert and does not react with food, which makes it an excellent choice for baking and storing food. The only problem with glass is that sudden temperature changes can cause breakage, so it is not suitable for use on the stovetop. Use glass for baking, mixing, and storing food.

Newer "clean" alternatives:

Titanium

Titanium is a slightly newer material used in cooking and has many of the same qualities as stainless steel. It is lightweight but may be cost prohibitive, as it tends to be more expensive than stainless.

Silicone

Silicone is generally considered safe because it is inert, heat resistant, and made from nontoxic compounds. However, it is essential to use high-quality silicone products and always follow the manufacturer's instructions. While we do use it for baking occasionally, it is not one of our go-to materials.

COOKWARE TO AVOID

This is the sneaky stuff that literally doesn't hold up under the heat. We recommend avoiding it almost exclusively.

Nonstick

Conventional nonstick cookware frequently includes perfluorooctanoic acid (PFOA) and polytetrafluoroethylene (PTFE). When exposed to elevated temperatures, these substances can emit fumes that might pose health risks if inhaled. The nonstick coating can easily scratch and deteriorate over time, potentially leaching harmful chemicals into food. It just doesn't stand the test of time, and we recommend steering clear of it—or replacing with clean cookware alternatives if you currently have nonstick cookware in your kitchen.

Aluminum

Lightweight, easy to use, and highly efficient at heat conductivity, aluminum is a popular cookware material, particularly in restaurants. The cause for concern with aluminum is primarily with acidic foods like tomatoes and vinegar. It also scratches and degrades over time. Excessive intake of aluminum has been associated with neurotoxicity.

What about aluminum foil? While generally considered safe, the concern with aluminum foil is using it to store acidic foods, and that it can become damaged with repeated use. We prefer parchment paper, because there is no risk of metal leaching and parchment is biodegradable.

Copper

Copper tends to be less popular because it is expensive, but copper cookware is excellent for even heat distribution, and it looks quite beautiful. However, prolonged exposure to high levels of copper can result in copper toxicity, as well as other adverse health effects. Nowadays, most copper cookware is lined with stainless steel, but it is important to double-check, and we would recommend that you avoid cooking with antique copper pots and pans. (But you can use them to decorate!)

Ceramic

Ceramic cookware is generally safe, but some products may contain heavy metals in their glazes. When using ceramics, it is important to consider the source and ask the manufacturer if you can. Unfortunately, heavy metals in glazes are a concern in vintage ceramics, and we would not recommend cooking with them. Most modern ceramicists use glazes that are safe to use unless noted otherwise.

In a world where virtually everything incites debate, we are not here to offer a one-size-fits-all prescription for wellness. We believe that there are many paths to a healthier life and that wellness is often deeply personal, defined by the cultures and customs we are familiar with. Much of feeling truly healthy in both mind and body is rooted in our attitude and intentions.

Ironically, the very pursuit of health can become unhealthy if we fixate on controlling every detail of our well-being, avoiding, or relentlessly chasing perfection. Instead, we hope to encourage a more balanced approach to caring for yourself and your family—one that blends logical, informed choices with a sense of ease and flexibility.

Ultimately, we aim to inspire you to feel empowered in your wellness journey, knowing that health is not just about rules but also about healthy routines, and living with intention, joy, and balance.

Now, let's eat!

The Recipes

Food is central to good health for us, not just because of its nutrients but because of its power to bring people together. When we sit down to eat with others, we're participating in a timeless ritual that can open up conversation, relax the nervous system, open our palate to other cultures, and ultimately create a sense of comfort and belonging—all essential aspects of holistic health. In this way, food serves as a foundation for better health, centralized on a ritual that can't be measured in nutrients alone.

We hope these recipes inspire you and get your own creative juices flowing. Don't think of recipes as rigid rules to follow; use them as a template or formula for learning more about how ingredients work together.

Use them, eat them, and share them! Now let's cook.

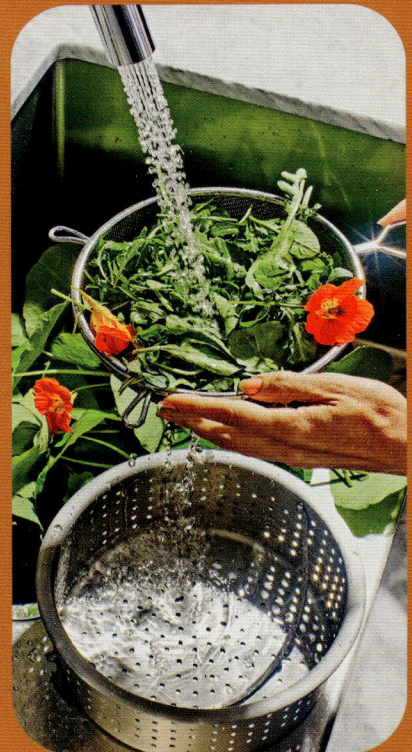

Help

Your

Self

Make Nut Milk

Making your own nut milks is so easy and doesn't require much time at all. There is a lot of information out there that makes it sound complicated, but it's really quite simple. Once you understand the ratio of nuts to water, feel free to try different combinations, flavors, and iterations: **See our suggested variations below.**

WHY SOAK?

The most practical reason for soaking is to soften the nuts and make them easier to blend, but there are some health benefits as well—soaking reduces phytic acid and enzyme inhibitors, which can reduce the bioavailability of nutrients and make them less easily digestible. It should be noted that these enzymes do not pose a significant issue for most people—if you're a busy person who forgot to soak your nuts (we've

been there!), then don't stress about it. And if you're in a rush, some nuts don't require any soaking at all. These are referred to in the chart below.

WHAT ARE ENZYME INHIBITORS?

The purpose of enzyme inhibitors in nature is to help the nut or seed avoid premature germination—they protect the seed until it is in the right conditions to sprout and grow into a plant. The two most common types of enzyme inhibitors are protease and amylase. Protease inhibitors block the enzyme that helps digest proteins, and amylase inhibitors impact the enzyme that breaks down carbohydrates. Again, for most people who do not suffer from digestive issues, these do not significantly impact the nutrient value or digestibility of nut milk.

NUT SOAKING CHART

NUTS	SOAK TIMES	NOTES
Almonds	6–8 hours	This is the standard soaking time, but overnight is best.
Hazelnuts	6–8 hours	Soaking overnight is recommended.
Walnuts	6–8 hours	Soaking is not necessary, but it does help remove bitter tannins.
Pecans	4–6 hours	Soft with a high fat content, so shorter soak times work well.
Brazil Nuts	4–6 hours	Typically on the softer side, so they require less soaking time. If you are short on time, soaking is not mandatory.
Cashews	1–2 hours	You don't need to soak cashews! They blend easily.
Macadamia Nuts	1–2 hours	Not necessary to soak, but soaking will yield creamier milk.
Pistachios	1–2 hours	Pistachios are soft and oily, so a shorter soak time is sufficient.
Sesame Seeds	1–2 hours	Soft, small, and oily, sesame seeds require minimal soaking.
Hemp Seeds	No soak	No soaking is necessary to make hemp milk.

DIY Better Nut Milk

MAKES ABOUT 4 CUPS (945 ML)

1 cup nuts (about 130 g)
(almonds, cashews, walnuts, and
pistachios are favorites)

Pinch sea salt

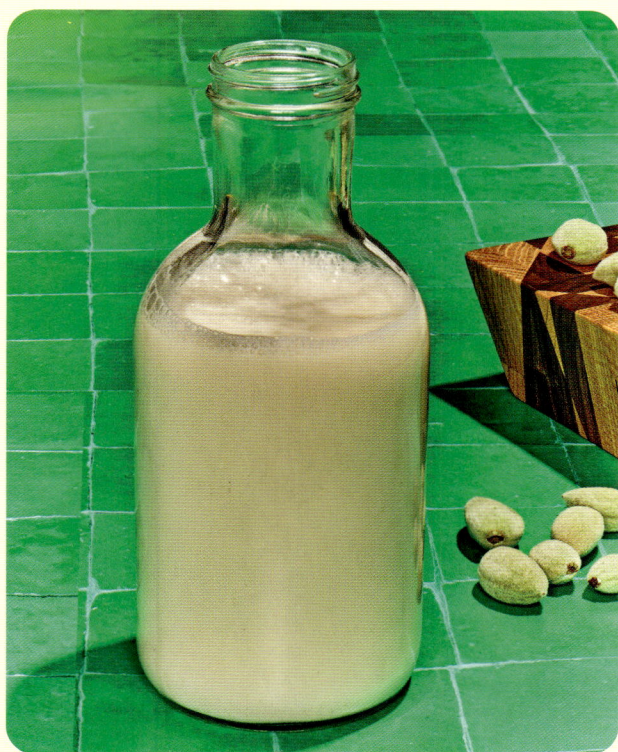

How to make?

The most common ratio for nut milk is 1:4, or 1 cup (about 130 g) nuts to every 4 cups (960 ml) water. If you prefer something creamier, then reduce the amount of water—or if you are looking to make a larger batch for cereal or oats, you can increase the water slightly.

Blend the nuts and sea salt with 4 cups (960 ml) water in a high-speed blender.

Strain through a nut milk bag or fine-mesh strainer, discarding the solids.

Serve immediately or refrigerate in an airtight container for up to 5 days.

* IF YOU OWN A HIGH-SPEED BLENDER, THESE SOAK TIMES CAN BE REDUCED BY HALF, BUT IF YOU ARE WORKING WITH A REGULAR BLENDER, WE RECOMMEND THE SOAK FOR EASE AND CREAMY RESULTS.

VARIATIONS

Coconut Butter
Adds a really nice creamy texture to the milk. One tablespoon for every cup (240 ml) water is enough to make a difference.

Coconut Oil
Use a little coconut oil in your milk—about 1 tablespoon per 4-cup (945 ml) batch—if you are looking to steam or froth it.

Honey
Adds a lovely sweetness, and also helps extend the shelf life of your milk to about 1 week.

Dates
Add 4 dates per 4 cup (32 oz) batch. This is our favorite whole food sweetening method because it just makes the milk taste so good.

Vanilla Extract
If you like vanilla-flavored milk, Add about 2 teaspoons per batch.

Spices
This is where you can get creative. We love cardamom, cinnamon, and turmeric. Add 1 teaspoon per 4 cup (32 oz) batch.

Help

Your

Self

Make Sauce

Having some great sauces in your repertoire is essential to making easy and versatile meals. The sauce recipes that follow can be used in rice dishes, on pasta, as salad dressings, dips . . . you name it.

Sauce making is an excellent opportunity to practice flavor balancing 101, because every sauce should include a sweet, salty, sour, and bitter element. Once you get the hang of it, the possible variations are endless—and can be so satisfying to make.

Our top two favorites are actually very different—the endlessly versatile nut butter sauce and a pesto-like sauce that uses a variety of nuts and herbs.

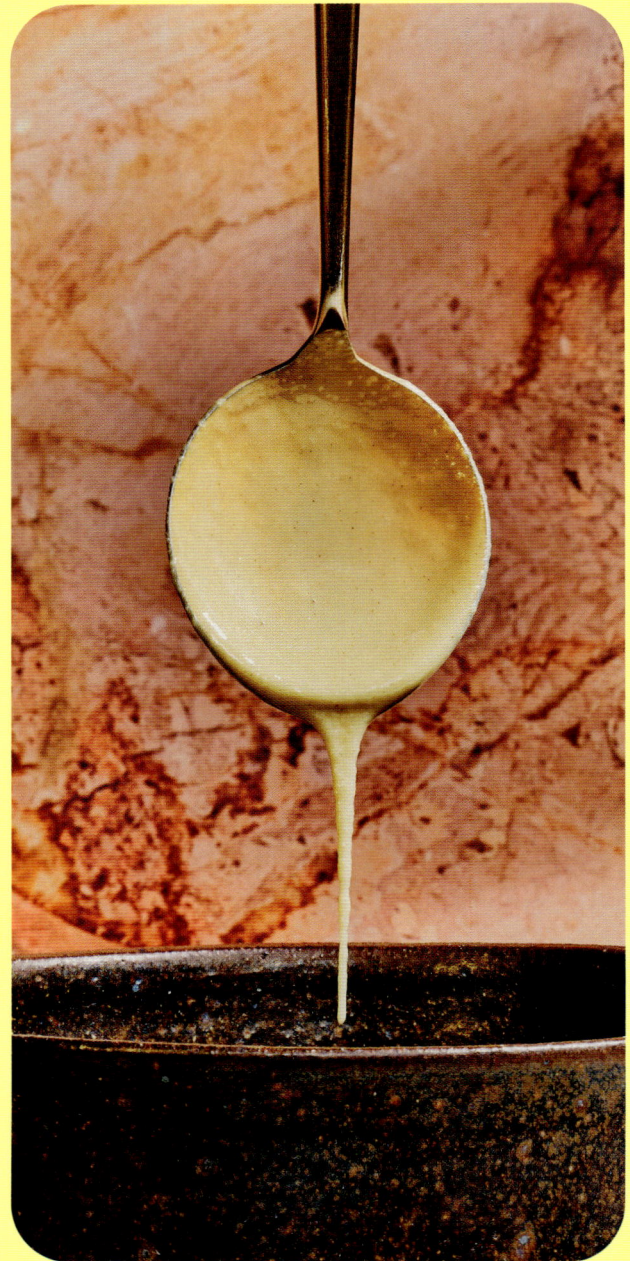

Better
Nut Butter
Sauce

MAKES ABOUT 1 CUP (240 ML)

½ cup (120 ml) nut butter (almond, cashew, and tahini are favorites)

2 tablespoons tamari or nama shoyu

2 tablespoons apple cider vinegar, rice vinegar, or fresh lemon juice

1 clove garlic (optional; mince if mixing in a bowl)

1 to 2 teaspoons chili paste or sriracha (optional)

Pinch sea salt

How to make?

In a bowl, blender, or food processor, whisk together or blend the nut butter, tamari, vinegar, garlic, if using, and chili paste, if you want some heat, until well combined.

Add ½ cup (120 ml) water, ¼ cup (60 ml) at a time, whisking or pulsing to achieve desired consistency. Add sea salt, taste, and adjust for seasoning.

Store in an airtight container in the refrigerator for up to 5 days.

VARIATIONS

Ginger
Great for digestion and a boost of flavor, fresh ginger is something we usually add. Finely mince it if you're whisking the sauce by hand.

Lime
Using lime instead of vinegar or lemon as the acid takes the sauce in an Asian-inspired direction.

Chives
Chopped chives as the allium are excellent instead of or in addition to the garlic.

Turmeric
Makes the sauce a beautiful yellow hue that brightens any dish.

Chopped Herbs
Add chopped herbs last, and get creative with your combos.

Chopped Nuts
To add texture and interest; this is the perfect addition when using the sauce as a dip.

All-Purpose Pesto

"Pesto" comes from the Italian word "pestare," meaning to crush or pound. For us, the contemporary version of this means putting our choice of pesto-like ingredients in a food processor (a full-size or mini food processor will work). Pulse it up into a paste and use it on everything.

Traditionally pesto is made from fresh basil, pine nuts, Parmesan cheese, garlic, and olive oil, but variations on the basic formula—provided below—are equally exciting and surprisingly nutrient-dense from all the herbs and healthy fats.

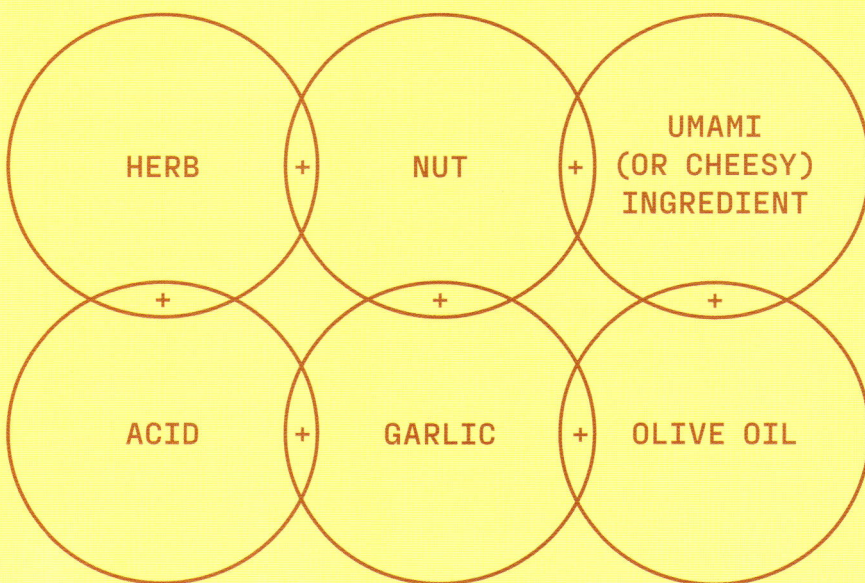

46

HERB + NUT + UMAMI (OR CHEESY) INGREDIENT

\+   +   +

ACID + GARLIC + OLIVE OIL

Cilantro Pumpkin Seed Pesto

Our favorite twist on the Italian version is this cilantro pesto using pumpkin seeds, but we've listed some of our other go-to variations on this recipe below.

MAKES ABOUT 1 CUP (240 ML)

2 cups (80 g) loosely packed fresh cilantro, including stems

½ cup (65 g) raw hulled pumpkin seeds

2 tablespoons white miso or nutritional yeast

2 cloves garlic

¼ cup (60 ml) fresh lemon juice

Pinch sea salt, or more to taste

½ cup (120 ml) olive oil

How to make?

Pulse the cilantro and pumpkin seeds in a food processor until the seeds are slightly broken up.

Add the miso, garlic, lemon juice, and sea salt. Pulse until well combined but make sure not to over-blend. Taste for salt.

Add the olive oil last and pulse until just combined. Store in an airtight container for up to 1 week.

TIP:
Please be mindful to add the oil last so that the pesto doesn't get sticky or gummy.

VARIATIONS

Walnut + Parsley
Swap in walnuts for the pumpkin seeds and parsley for the cilantro. Delicious served on mushrooms, beets, and other heartier fare.

Basil + Lime
Substitute basil for the cilantro and lime juice for the lemon. Add 1 teaspoon red pepper flakes. Great on rice noodles or tofu, or in curries.

Pistachio + Lemon
Use basil or cilantro as the herb, pistachio as the nut, and add 1 tablespoon lemon zest.

Arugula
Use arugula instead of an herb. Excellent on any pasta, it adds a nice spicy kick that will turn up the flavor of just about anything.

Olive
Use cured olives in place of the nuts, to create more of a tapenade that is very rich and briny in flavor. You can reduce the amount of olive oil by ¼ cup (60 ml).

Romesco
Pulse together 1 cup (55 g) sun-dried tomatoes, 1 cup (140 g) roasted red pepper, ½ cup (70 g) almonds, and 2 teaspoons dried herbs like basil, parsley, or thyme, along with olive oil. We love this version served on toast or in sandwiches.

Help

Your

Self

Make Beans

For some reason making beans from scratch is an overwhelming prospect for many people, but getting the hang of making a fresh pot is truly a life-changing experience and facilitates making an endless array of healthy meals. Use beans in a grain bowl, on salads, mashed as a dip, tossed in pasta, or crisped up in the oven as a crunchy snack.

As you'll see from the chart below, if you start soaking beans in water at the beginning of the day, most varieties will cook in about 45 minutes, depending on the freshness of the beans (fresher = faster), for a healthy dinner with very little active time involved.

TIPS:

● **Quick soak:** To reduce the soaking time of any bean, you can boil the water for 2 to 3 minutes before soaking. This will make the soak time approximately 1 to 2 hours for any bean.

● **Soaking times:** If you miss your timer or need to get dinner started early, don't fret. A little longer or a little shorter won't make a huge difference in the end result.

● **Salting:** There is some controversy around when to salt beans for optimal texture: before, during, or at the end of cooking. We typically salt after soaking and once the water starts to boil.

● **Adding acid:** If you're looking to add tomatoes or vinegar, wait and do this toward the end of cooking. If you add acid too early, it can hinder the cooking process.

● **Storage:** After they've cooled to room temperature, cooked beans can be stored in an airtight container in the refrigerator for 4 to 5 days or in the freezer for up to 2 months.

BEAN COOKING CHART

BEAN TYPE	SOAKING TIME	COOKING TIME	NOTES
Almonds	6–8 hours	45–60 minutes	Aka turtle beans
Black-Eyed Peas	4–6 hours	40–50 minutes	Soaking isn't required
Cannellini Beans	6–8 hours	45–60 minutes	Aka white kidney beans
Chickpeas	8–12 hours	1–2 hours	Aka garbanzo beans
Kidney Beans	6–8 hours	1–1½ hours	Super meaty
Lima Beans	6–8 hours	1–1½ hours	Try Christmas limas
Navy Beans	6–8 hours	1–1½ hours	Small, good in soup
Pinto Beans	6–8 hours	1–1½ hours	Use for refried beans
Soybeans	8–12 hours	2–3 hours	Longest to cook
Lentils	No soaking	20–30 minutes	Lentils cook fast

The Best Beans

1 pound (455 g) dry beans (about 2 cups) of your choice

2- to 4-inch (5 to 10 cm) piece of kombu seaweed (optional, but used traditionally in Japan to increase digestibility of beans by reducing phytic acid)

Aromatics of your choice (2 cloves garlic, ½ onion, or a few bay leaves)

Sea salt

How to make?

Place beans in a bowl and cover with room-temperature water by 1 to 2 inches (2.5 to 5 cm). Let soak according to the time specified in the chart opposite, then drain the beans.

Add the soaked beans to a medium-large saucepan and cover with water by 1 to 2 inches (2.5 to 5 cm). You want the beans to be fully submerged in water. Add the seaweed, if using, along with aromatics of your choice. Save salt for the end of cooking.

Bring the beans to a boil over medium-high heat. Reduce the heat and simmer for the cook time specified in the chart opposite, partially covering the pot to reduce evaporation. Stir every 10 minutes or so just to keep an eye on things, but the beans will cook themselves. Add salt within the last 20 minutes of cooking. Add any spices, or vegetable variations, during the last 10 minutes of cooking.

Check for doneness by pricking the beans with a fork, starting at the low end of the cook-time range. You want them to pierce easily without being mushy. Taste and adjust for salt and other flavoring. Yes, it's that easy.

Got bean juice?

Our last note on beans will be about the lovely liquid that gets produced during the bean cooking process. This liquid gold of bean cooking is called aquafaba. Aquafaba can be used as an egg substitute in vegan baking and desserts, to thicken dressings, and in pretty much any recipe that calls for egg whites.

The most commonly used aquafaba comes from cooking chickpeas (the color and flavor is the most versatile), but any bean juice will work.

If you're not inclined to use bean juice as an egg replacement, this leftover liquid can be used as a wholesome and flavorful substitute for broth in any recipe.

VARIATIONS

Bean Hummus
In a blender, combine 2 cups (370 g) cooked beans, ¼ cup (60 ml) tahini, ¼ cup (60 ml) fresh lemon juice, and 1 clove garlic and blend until smooth. Add 2 tablespoons olive oil and salt to taste and pulse to combine.

Bean Salad
Add ½ cup (90 g) beans per serving to any salad.

Bean Pâte
In a food processor, combine 2 cups (370 g) cooked beans, ½ cup (50 g) walnuts, 1 clove garlic, 1 tablespoon fresh lemon juice, 1 teaspoon sea salt, and olive oil and fresh herbs to taste. Pulse to a texture that is smooth and velvety or coarse and hearty, depending on your preference.

Pasta with Beans
Add 2 cups (370 g) cooked beans to any pasta dish.

Crispy Beans
Toss beans in olive oil and season generously with sea salt. We like to add ½ teaspoon turmeric powder and ½ teaspoon chili powder, but try different spices and herbs of your liking. Spread evenly on a baking sheet and bake in a preheated 400°F (205°C) oven for 20 to 30 minutes. Shake the baking sheet halfway through to ensure that the beans cook evenly. Enjoy as a salad topper or on their own.

Help

Your

Self

Make Grains

Grains, especially whole grains, are the foundation for many of the meals prepared in our households—both lunch and dinner. If you've never used a rice cooker, we highly recommend trying one, as they can be used to make any type of grain, not just rice.

Whole grains are a foundational ingredient for good health. Although they have a complicated rap here in the US, they are a staple food for the healthiest cultures in the world.

Whole grains make all the difference; they are rich in fiber, high in B vitamins, and deliver essential minerals like iron, magnesium, and zinc. The refining process depletes grains of essential nutrients, leaving behind an inferior, less nourishing product.

"I typically forgo the perfect texture of the *set it and forget it* rice cooker method, and to be totally honest, I typically use a 1:2 ratio for almost every grain. But, if you're more diligent than me, follow the chart below and the directions for stovetop grains that make life super tasty."

—MEREDITH

GRAIN COOKING CHART

GRAIN TYPE	GRAIN-TO-LIQUID RATIO	COOKING TIME
Rice (White, Long Grain)	1:2	15–20 minutes
Rice (Brown)	1:2.5	40–45 minutes
Rice (Basmati, Jasmine)	1:1.5	15–20 minutes
Quinoa	1:2	15–20 minutes
Couscous (Traditional)	1:1.5	5 minutes
Bulgur	1:2	12–15 minutes
Barley	1:3	40–50 minutes
Millet	1:2.5	20–25 minutes
Farro	1:2.5	25–35 minutes
Spelt	1:3	1–1½ hours
Oats (Rolled)	1:2	5–10 minutes
Oats (Steel-Cut)	1:4	25–30 minutes

The Perfect Grains

MAKES ABOUT 3 CUPS (555 G)

1 cup (185 g) of your preferred grain
(we like to mix it up on the regular)

2 cups (480 ml) liquid (water, dashi,
or veggie broth)

1 tablespoon olive or avocado oil (optional)

Pinch sea salt

OPTIONAL:

1 clove garlic, minced

1-inch (2.5 cm) chunk of ginger

½ teaspoon turmeric powder or 1-inch (2.5 cm) piece
fresh turmeric, grated

Dried spices: ½ teaspoon cumin, coriander, cinnamon,
cardamom, or paprika, to name a few of our favorites

How to make?

Rinse the grain under cold water to remove any dust or
excess starch. Drain well.

Add oil, if using. If you are using any aromatics like onions,
garlic, ginger, turmeric, or other spices, sauté them before
adding to the grain for deeper flavor.

Add the grain to a saucepan or skillet. Cover the grain with
the liquid (water or broth), add the sea salt, and stir.

Bring to a boil over medium-high heat. Once the liquid
boils, reduce heat to low. Cover the pan with a lid and let
it simmer. Cook times vary based on grain, so refer to the
chart opposite for approximate cooking time.

Taste for doneness. You want to make sure the grain is soft
without being mushy. Once cooked, remove from heat and
fluff with a fork before serving. Store in an airtight container in the refrigerator for up to 1 week.

VARIATIONS

Herby Grains
Add about 1 loosely packed cup
(50 g) of your favorite chopped
herbs plus 2 tablespoons olive
oil and an extra pinch of sea salt
to room-temperature grains.

Spanish Style
Our favorite! Add 1 small diced
onion, 1 clove garlic, and 1 cup
(240 ml) tomato sauce to the
grain when adding the liquid.
Stir well to combine and cook
according to the directions
provided.

Turmeric Coconut
Add 1 tablespoon coconut
oil and 1 tablespoon turmeric
powder to the grains when
you add the liquid and cook as
described.

Vegetables
Incorporate diced vegetables
like bell peppers, carrots, and
zucchini, and fresh herbs. You
can sauté them before adding
to the grain, or add as a raw
addition. Include extra salt and
olive oil.

Beans
The addition of 2 cups cooked
beans (370 g) to 1 cup (175 g)
cooked grain is excellent in all
combinations.

Citrus
Add 2 tablespoons lemon or
lime juice and 1 tablespoon
citrus zest at the end of
cooking, plus a pinch of sea
salt.

Pesto
Toss cooked grains with pesto;
serve with beans and greens.

Salad
Add grains to any greens and
finish with a simple salad
dressing such as our Better
Nut Butter Sauce (page 45)
with tahini.

BUILD YOUR BOWL

Grain
+
Green
+
Sauce
+
Any vegetables
of your choice

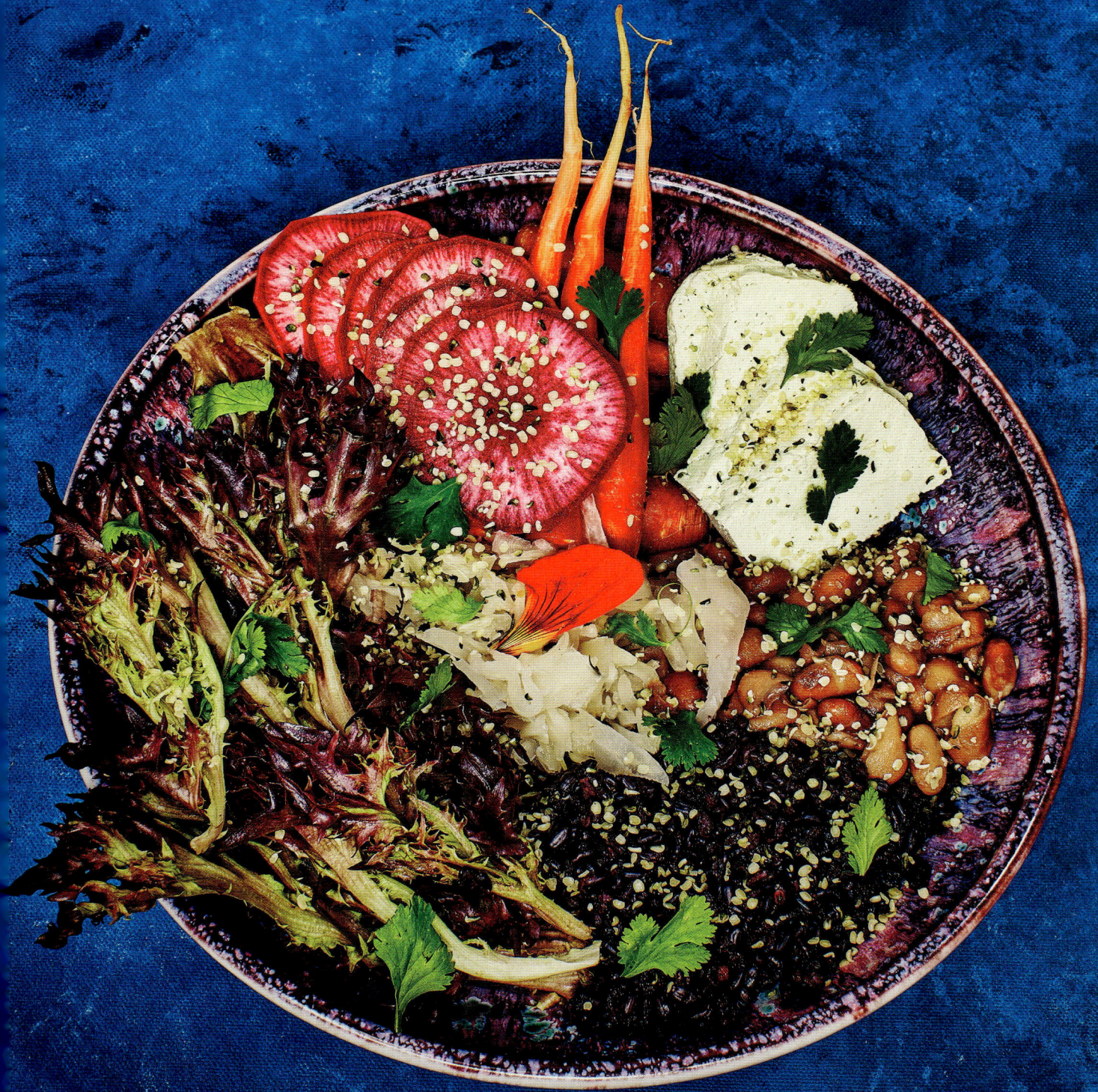

Love

"

I had terrible digestion in my early years and as a teenager. I remember visiting family and discussing "digestion" in front of my uncle, who was a gastroenterologist. He said that in forty years of practice, I talked more about digestive health than anyone he'd ever met. This was in the nineties, when the connection between gut health, mental health, and overall well-being was essentially poo-pooed by mainstream science (pun intended). But as the years passed, and I learned more about gut health and its importance, science started to back up what I'd always known to be true. I'm happy to say I've had great digestion for years, and science now supports my antics.
—MEREDITH

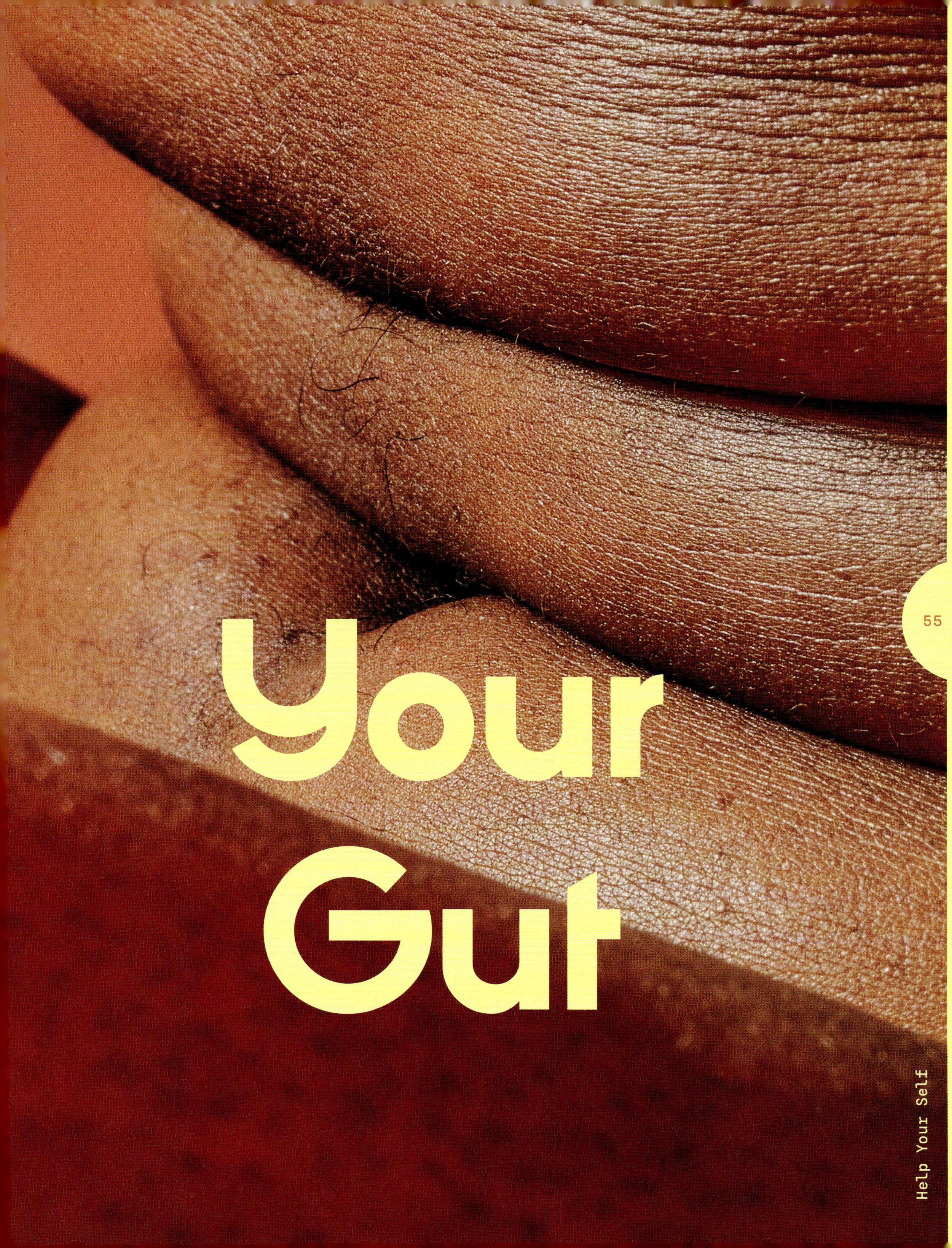

Your Gut

Gut health, as defined in this chapter, refers to the balance and function of bacteria throughout the entire gastrointestinal tract. It reflects how well our digestive system processes food, absorbs nutrients, and eliminates waste. This balance influences everything from digestion and nutrient absorption to immune function, mental health, and even skin health.

We believe gut health and understanding the function of your microbiome are among the most critical aspects of overall health and well-being.

56

If your gut health isn't in check, you probably aren't well hydrated, you won't sleep well, your mood and stress levels will be impacted, your skin health will suffer, and none of that will lead to a great sex life. Therefore, in our book, it all goes back to the gut.

Statistically, around 16 percent of the US population is affected by constipation and gut health issues. As we get older, the chances of experiencing these issues increase, and women (probably due to hormones) more commonly suffer from constipation than men. And as if feeling backed up (or the opposite) isn't bad enough, because of the gut-brain connection, gut issues can trigger—and be caused by—anxiety, stress, and depression.

This is why gut microbiome health is essential—it's really the new frontier of health. We want to give you the lowdown on how it works, so that you can start optimizing your digestion to feel better physically and mentally. Concepts in this chapter include maintaining a healthy gut, proper elimination, optimal feeding cycles, fiber intake, and more.

As the kids' book says, everybody poops. So, let's normalize talking about it, rather than making it a taboo or stressful topic.

Microbiome Basics

Most of us have heard about the importance of the gut microbiome, but we may not fully understand it. We're here to help.

What is the microbiome?

Time for a little science lesson. The human body is populated by trillions of microorganisms, mostly bacteria, but also fungi, viruses, and their genes, which make up the microbiome. We have collections of these microorganisms, called microbiota, in every part of our body, but the collection in our gut appears most numerous and most important for human health. Microbial diversity in the gut is super important for health—but many of us don't have it, and we'll get to why that is in this chapter.[1]

A diverse range of microbiota in our gut is crucial for carrying out the following functions:

→ **Supporting digestion.** "Good" gut bacteria break our food down, delivering essential nutrients to the body and supporting metabolic processes.

→ **Maintaining the integrity of our intestinal barrier.** You've probably heard of "leaky gut," which occurs when gut disruption causes undigested food particles and toxins to leak into the bloodstream, leading to inflammation.

→ **Regulating our immune system and protecting against disease.** By outcompeting harmful microbes and modulating the immune system, the microbiome can respond more efficiently to infections.

→ **Modulating our weight.** Studies have linked lower bacterial diversity in the gut with obesity.[2]

57

The long and short of it is that when there is a lack of microbial diversity in the gut, these functions are disrupted, leading to a cascade of resulting health problems.

How does our microbiome develop?

The human microbiome is an ever-evolving ecosystem shaped by numerous factors.

Our microbes originate from various sources and will continually change throughout our lives, improving or declining in diversity. This begins with how we're born, whether via vaginal delivery or C-section. It continues with the environmental factors we're exposed to (like where we live and whether we own pets), and the choices that we make about diet, hygiene practices, and our social interactions (like being around germy children). All these factors play a role in microbiome composition.

Microbes are everywhere and we're exposed to them constantly. So, what's the problem? Well, over the last fifty years, several factors have reduced our exposure to microbial diversity, leading to gut imbalance.

While some of these factors have had benefits for our health, they have also impacted the gut bacteria of the average modern human quite significantly:

The Processed Western Diet

The typical Western or Standard American Diet is linked to reduced microbial diversity primarily due to a need for more fiber, limited consumption of fermented foods, and a reliance on ultra-processed foods. Foods that are processed are so far removed from their natural state that our bodies often struggle to break them down properly, depriving our gut bacteria, and our whole bodies, of essential nutrients. Additionally, processed foods are often full of refined sugar, which promotes the growth of less beneficial bacteria, and leads to an imbalance in the microbial ecosystem.

Widespread Antibiotic Use

"Antibiotics can be lifesaving, and we absolutely do not stand against using them at all. However, we believe in limiting our exposure by choosing foods that are produced without them; not always relying on them as the first line of defense during illness (with doctor supervision); and being mindful of supplementing with a round of probiotics after any truly necessary antibiotic course. We advocate for awareness, not avoidance."

—MEREDITH

When you are sick, or when your kids are sick, you want to knock that bug out as quickly as possible. And you should always seek the advice of a medical professional. However, requesting a prescription for antibiotics at your doctor's office may not always be the way to go. Early-life antibiotic exposure may reduce microbial diversity and delay the normal development of the gut microbiome, leading to an increased risk of developing allergies, asthma, type 1 diabetes, and obesity later in childhood.[3]

Of course, antibiotics can be lifesaving, and we're not saying to avoid them. But we'd advise taking them judiciously as needed and replenishing your gut bacteria with probiotics after an antibiotic course. The overprescription of antibiotics is not the only issue here. Studies also show that the consumption of animal products treated with antibiotics can affect the quality of your microbiome.[4] When shopping for meat, eggs, or dairy, look for labels that specifically note "raised without antibiotics."

Hygiene and Our Over-Sanitized Environments

We're all for hand washing, and while stringent hygiene practices effectively curb the spread of infectious diseases, they may limit our exposure to various beneficial microorganisms. But it's not just hand washing that poses an issue—it's the use of harsh cleansers and the overuse of hand sanitizer and antibacterial soaps, which have their place in killing bad bacteria. And, unless you are truly buying everything at a farmers' market (or growing your own food—we're not!), be aware that most supermarket food has been cleaned and sprayed so thoroughly that it lacks the beneficial microbes from the soil it came from.

The Rise of C-Sections

During a vaginal birth, a baby's gut microbiome is colonized by microbes from their mother's vaginal and fecal flora. This transfer does not occur during a birth via C-section, which initially results in a less diverse microbiome for the baby. It has been reported that babies born by C-section are more likely to develop allergies, asthma, and future metabolic complications.[5]

However, let's keep in mind that a safe, healthy birth for both baby and mother is what's most important. We share these facts not to cause fear or frustration, especially if you're a mother who delivered via C-section. We want to arm you with knowledge, because there's a lot you can do to support a baby's microbiome post-birth or to recolonize your own gut microbiome for improved health. We're going to give you the tools in this chapter.

Urban Living

Urban landscapes, with their concrete jungles and limited access to nature, often deprive people of exposure to the rich array of microorganisms found in rural environments. Even if you don't live in an urban setting, the increase in time spent indoors and living from home to car to office, with limited interaction with the natural world, can hurt your gut health. So, get out there and spend some time digging in the dirt, take a hike, or get a pet, all of which will increase your exposure to a diverse range of microbes.

The F word

When it comes to restoring and preserving gut health in the modern world, the F word is key. Yes, you guessed it—fiber. Fiber regulates the gut microbiota, creating an environment for healthy bacteria to flourish.[6] You may also be interested to know that fiber is a carbohydrate found only in plant-based foods—fruits, vegetables, grains, beans, and greens. Unlike other carbohydrates that break down into sugars, fiber passes through the digestive system relatively intact, effectively scrubbing the colon clean of unnecessary waste and matter.

We've got a fiber problem.

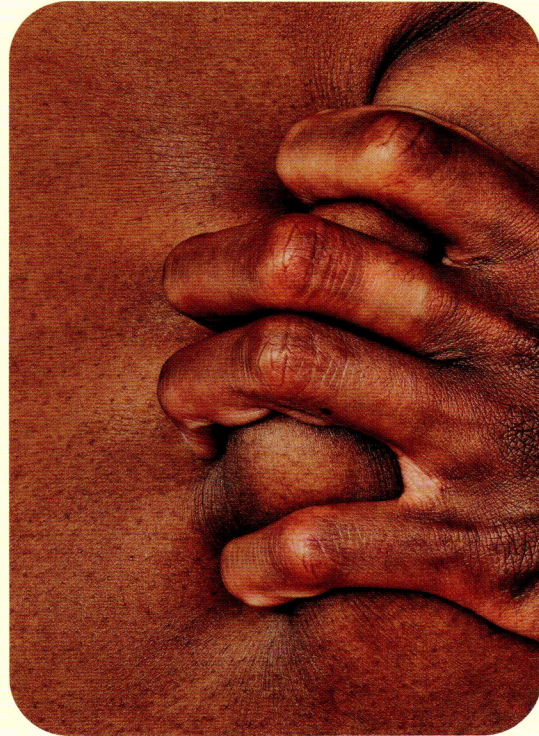

The average American consumes only about 16 grams of fiber daily, falling significantly short of the recommended minimum of 25 to 38 grams. This deficit is primarily because the American diet is loaded with processed and refined foods, with a low intake of fruits, vegetables, whole grains, and legumes. The implications are substantial, leading to chronic issues such as constipation, high cholesterol, poor blood sugar control, heightened risks of heart disease, obesity, and possibly certain cancers.

Fiber is crucial to our health for the following reasons:

DIGESTIVE HEALTH

High-fiber foods help bulk up stool and promote regular bowel movements, preventing constipation and helping to regulate digestive health. Fiber helps to keep the digestive system running smoothly, which can reduce strain on the intestines and prevent inflammation. If you think of digestive health as the plumbing, fiber is the pipe cleaner.

GUT HEALTH

Gut health differs from digestive health, even though the two work very much in tandem—if one is off, the other likely will be, too. While "digestive health" refers to digestion and excretion, "gut health" is the functionality of the inner tube food moves through, from the stomach to the intestines and colon. Fiber is crucial to gut health because it acts as a prebiotic, feeding the beneficial gut bacteria that is essential for a healthy digestive system. If we stick to our plumbing analogy, the gut is like the drain or disposal system. If it is clogged, or not functioning properly, everything will get backed up.

BLOOD SUGAR CONTROL

Fiber slows the digestion and absorption of sugar, helping maintain steady blood sugar levels and preventing spikes. Slower digestion leads to more blood sugar regulation, and fewer cravings and out-of-control hunger pangs.[7]

MAINTAINING CHOLESTEROL AND HEART HEALTH

Fiber can help reduce LDL, or "bad" cholesterol, by binding to cholesterol particles in the digestive system, preventing their absorption from food and reabsorbtion from bile, and moving them out of the system.[8] In addition to aiding in the removal of cholesterol, high-fiber diets can also help lower blood pressure and reduce inflammation, improving cardiovascular health.

WEIGHT MANAGEMENT

When we consume high-fiber foods, the bulk they add to our diet takes longer to digest, providing a sustained release of energy and preventing rapid spikes and drops in blood sugar levels that can trigger hunger. In contrast, foods that are low in fiber tend to be digested quickly, leading to a rapid return of hunger and an increased likelihood of overeating.

These are our top five ways to get more fiber into your diet:

(1) INCORPORATE WHOLE GRAINS

"To grain or not to grain" seems to forever be a dietary question, but we 100% support eating more whole grains. Science has shown time and time again the value of eating a high-fiber diet, and whole grains are a great way to do it.

(2) SNACK SMART

The snack world has gotten super complicated, and we advise keeping it simple. Look to fruits, vegetables, nuts, and other high-fiber foods. In our opinion, an apple with some almond butter is the queen of the snack landscape: endlessly portable, satisfying crunch, tastes good—and helps clean your teeth! (Through the natural scrubbing and malic acid that gently removes stains.) Although we generally advise limited snacking, approaching it mindfully through healthy choices is the key.

(3) ADD BEANS AND LEGUMES

Whether you're on an entirely veggie path or not, beans are one of the richest sources of fiber of all foods, and this includes not only black, kidney, and navy beans, but also lentils, chick-peas, and peas.

(4) SPRINKLE SOME SEEDS

Again, no matter what you eat, sprinkling any dish with seeds (sunflower, pumpkin, sesame, and hemp are some of our faves) is a great way to get more fiber and elevate your food presentation at the same time!

(5) ADD AVOCADO

This might be the easiest suggestion. Not only is adding avocado a great way to boost flavor and appeal (and healthy fat), but it's also high in fiber.

Migrating Motor Complex (MMC)

We've covered fiber. Now let's cut to an even sexier topic: Migrating Motor Complex (MMC), which is all about the importance of letting your digestive system rest to digest.

There is so much emphasis placed on what to eat, but we'd like to come right out and say that the number one thing you can do to boost overall gut health is to improve your resting digestion. A healthy diet will only get you so far if you're not giving your digestive system a chance to rest. The MMC is like a cleansing wave that happens during digestion to move food residue from the small intestine into the colon, acting as an intestinal housekeeper.

62

A properly functioning MMC uses its housekeeper function to prevent bacterial overgrowth in the upper gastrointestinal tract, regulates hunger and satiety, and aids in nutrient absorption. Problems occur when the MMC isn't working properly, and food stays in the stomach and intestine longer than is healthy, leading to all kinds of problems.

The Four Phases of MMC

The MMC consists of the following four phases, which repeat every 90 to 120 minutes:

→ PHASE I
A period of inactivity lasting 30 to 60 minutes.

→ PHASE II
A period of intermittent contractions that gradually increase in intensity and frequency, lasting about 20 to 40 minutes.

→ PHASE III
A short burst of regular, intense contractions (called the "housekeeper wave") that sweep through the stomach and small intestine, lasting about 10 to 20 minutes.

→ PHASE IV
A brief transition period back to Phase I, lasting 10 to 15 minutes.

So how do we support our MMC and improve our resting digestion? We recommend the following:

- **Limit snacking and eliminate grazing.**
Backed by science, and confirmed by personal experience, we want to tell you that snacking in excess can wreck your digestive system. Many people don't eat proper meals but will rely on constant snacking to manage nutrient intake. Not only is this not great for weight management, but it can also mess with your digestion. Taking breaks between meals is vital for good digestion. Allow your MMC to do its work by fasting between meals and snacks, aiming for a three- to four-hour window when you are not eating. We recognize that sometimes a snack is essential for an energy boost, or to stave off hunger—this is when it's time to snack smartly. However, the endless snack, or "grazing," is when we get into digestive trouble.

- **Incorporate fasting periods.**
You should aim to give your MMC a break for 8 to 12 hours between dinner and breakfast.

- **Stay hydrated.**
We will talk more about this in Chapter 4: Help Your Self Hydrate (page 118), but proper hydration is essential in improving our digestion and supporting the MMC by ensuring smooth and effective gut mobility.

- **Reduce stress.**
This is easier said than done, and we'll address stress management in Chapter 6: Help Your Self Stress Less (page 168), but not eating when actively stressed is a good rule of thumb for improving digestion. (Many people do the opposite, we know.)

- **Take probiotics.**
Taking probiotic supplements regularly is scientifically proven to help with digestive issues. If you are regularly eating food-based probiotics (such as yogurt, sauerkraut, kimchi, natto, etc.) and experiencing efficient digestion, it is possible to reduce probiotic supplement consumption to an as-needed basis.

When is the best time to eat?

According to science, the best way to eat for optimal gut health, digestion, and weight management is to limit your window for eating. We've all heard of intermittent fasting at this point, but we find that term to be slightly misleading. It isn't so much about fasting as it is about reducing the window in which you eat.

For example, if you eat breakfast at 6 a.m. and dinner at 9 p.m., that is a fifteen-hour window, which is a long one. But if breakfast is at 10 a.m. and dinner is at 6 p.m., that's a much shorter, eight-hour window, increasing the amount of time that you aren't eating and allowing for digestion and nutrient absorption. The science behind this is based on the function of the MMC and the time spent between meals to increase the efficacy of digestion.

Breaking the fast?

Breakfast is often touted as the most important meal of the day, but this belief isn't universally true. As long as you eat enough calories throughout the day, skipping breakfast can extend your digestive rest window. Emerging research suggests that the significance of breakfast depends on individual metabolism, lifestyle, and preferences. Do you wake up hungry? Then you might be someone who metabolically thrives on breakfast. Some people thrive on intermittent fasting or eating later in the day without an early meal. Furthermore, the idea that breakfast is essential for weight management or productivity is increasingly being challenged, as what truly matters is the overall quality of one's diet and aligning eating patterns with personal needs.

> "Hydration and elimination are always the emphasis for me in the morning. Once elimination has occurred, then it is time for breakfast. I personally believe that this should be the standard for most people. The idea that 'breakfast is the most important meal of the day,' or that it must be eaten right when you wake up, has its roots in various marketing, historical, and cultural influences that are not necessarily applicable to the modern world. I would never recommend starting your day hungry or with low blood sugar, but most people would benefit from hydration, movement, and elimination before eating their first meal. You have to listen to your body first."
>
> —MEREDITH

The Gut-Brain Connection

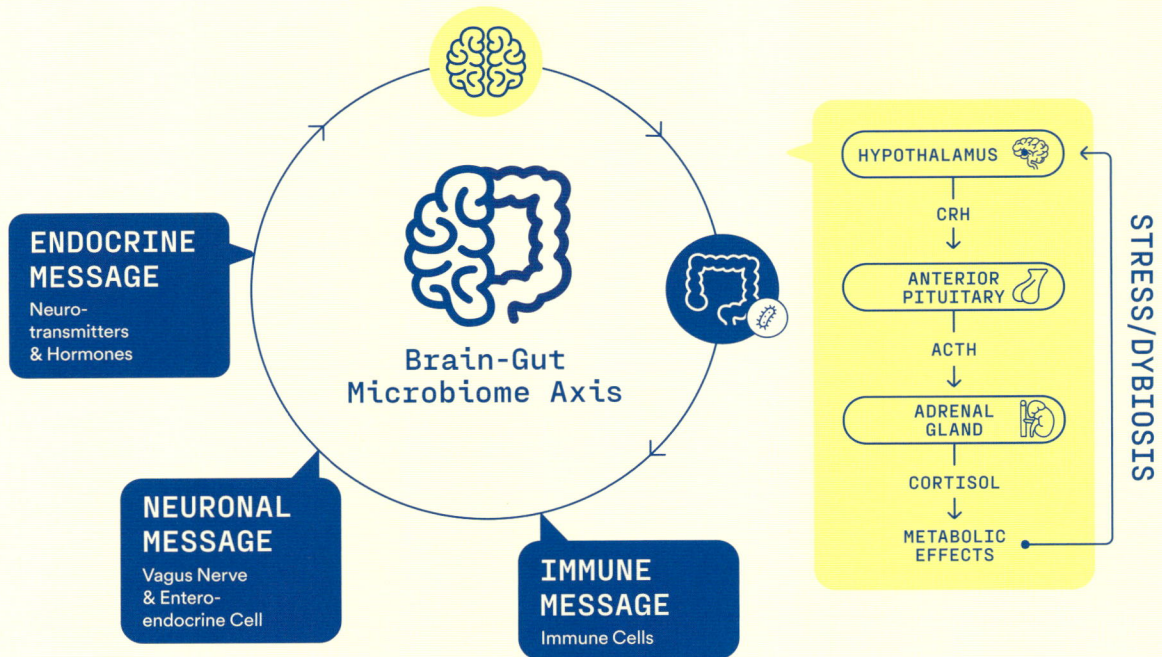

ENDOCRINE MESSAGE

Neuro-transmitters & Hormones

Brain-Gut Microbiome Axis

NEURONAL MESSAGE

Vagus Nerve & Entero-endocrine Cell

IMMUNE MESSAGE

Immune Cells

HYPOTHALAMUS

CRH

ANTERIOR PITUITARY

ACTH

ADRENAL GLAND

CORTISOL

METABOLIC EFFECTS

STRESS/DYBIOSIS

"I know that my gut health has a major effect on my mental health. I used to suffer from constipation, and it significantly increased my anxiety and stress levels. I think having poor digestion can also affect your relationship to food and make it harder to navigate food cravings, signals, and satiety. I still get crabby if I'm constipated, which fortunately rarely happens."

—MEREDITH

The connection between gut health and brain health is a topic of conversation in the wellness world that is finally getting the mainstream attention it deserves. Not only is poor gut health uncomfortable, but it can have a considerable impact on mental health conditions, ranging from mild to severe.[9]

This is all thanks to what scientists call the Gut-Brain Axis, which is a two-way communication network that links the central nervous system (the brain) and the enteric nervous system (the gastrointestinal tract). This complex system involves multiple pathways, including neural, hormonal, and immunological mechanisms, that allow for constant back-and-forth communication between the gut and the brain.

Here are some of the ways that gut-brain communication happens along these pathways:

CORTISOL

When we are stressed, the body produces the "stress hormone" cortisol, which directly affects gut function. There are cortisol receptors in various gut cells, and when cortisol is released, it can cause intestinal permeability or "leaky gut," allowing harmful bacteria and toxins to enter the bloodstream.

SEROTONIN

Serotonin, aka "the happiness hormone," has been established as a significant contributor to brain-gut conditions.[10] Most of the serotonin we produce is absorbed in the intestine, and a deficiency of serotonin in the central nervous system (CNS) is a crucial factor contributing to depression, sadness, and anxiety. It is currently understood as a primary cause of depressed mood or depression.[11]

VAGUS NERVE

The vagus nerve is a bidirectional nerve that connects the gut to the brain, allowing microbes to send signals to the brain. Changes in gut bacteria can stimulate the vagus nerve, which may reduce stress and anxiety. Early research also shows that stimulating the vagus nerve may help with treatment-resistant depression, PTSD, and inflammatory bowel disease.[12]

HORMONES

More than thirty gut hormone genes are expressed and found in the gastrointestinal tract, making it the body's largest endocrine (hormonal) organ. Anticipating a meal or having food in the upper gastrointestinal tract triggers the release of gut hormones and neurotransmitters. Gut hormones, regulated by gut microbiota, are essential for sending signals about nutrition and energy from the gut to the brain to help regulate food intake and appetite.[13]

IMMUNE FUNCTION

Damage to the gut lining can lead to intestinal inflammation, which regulates immune function. Factors such as a Western diet, antibiotic use, and stress can negatively affect the gut lining, allowing bacteria and other foreign particles to enter and trigger an immune response.[14]

Gut-brain health is a two-way process; one regulates the other. Understanding the gut-brain axis is crucial for developing new treatments for various conditions, from gastrointestinal disorders to mental health issues. This highlights the importance of a holistic approach to health that considers the intricate connections between the gut and the brain.

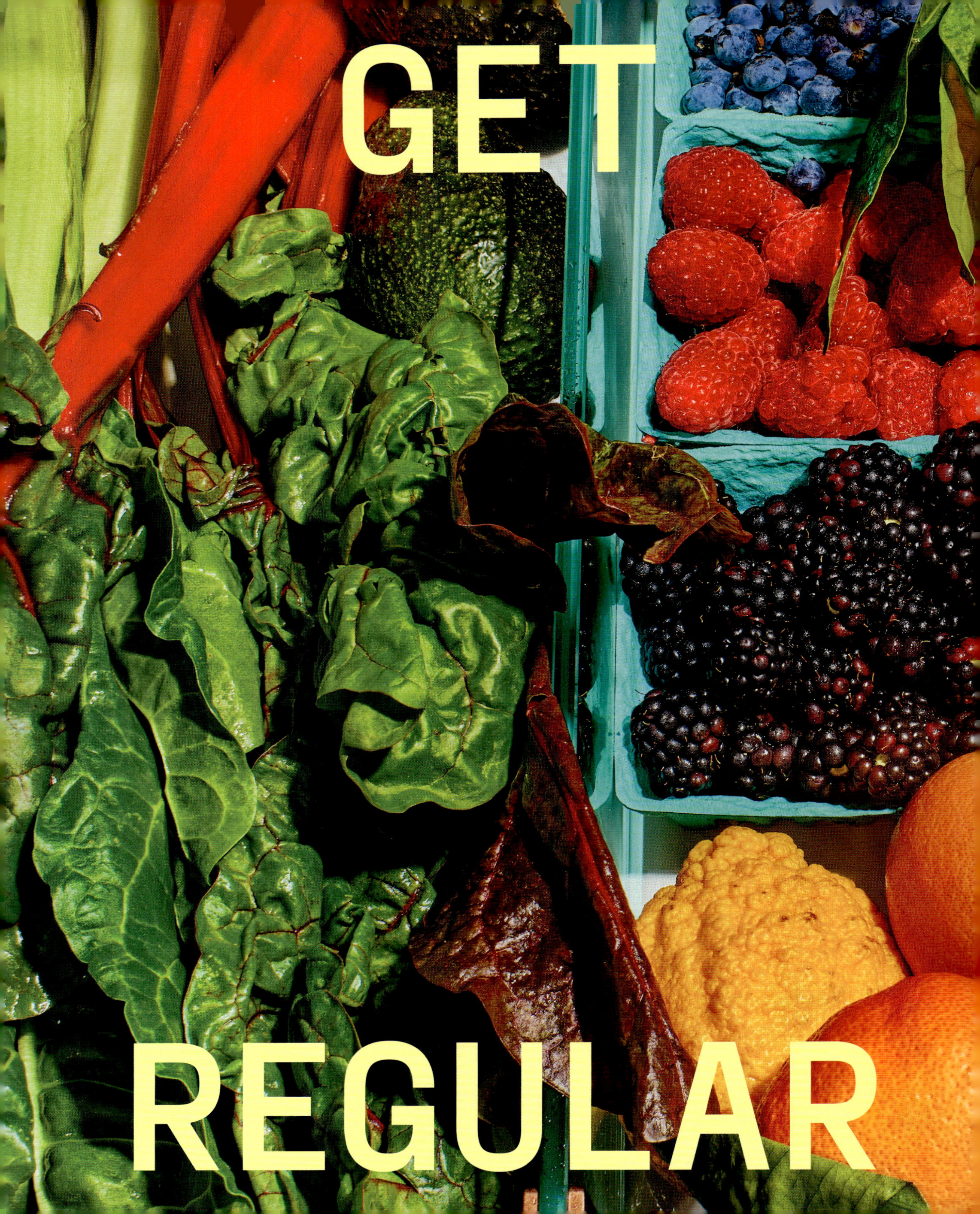

GET

REGULAR

" When I first met my husband, I shamelessly told him that I must be left alone in the mornings: Don't talk to me or look at me until I've digested. I rely on coffee and a big glass of water to get things moving. It wasn't always so easy for me, but after years of suffering from subpar digestion and constipation, I can now say (knock on wood) that I have my routine figured out. Read on for how you too can experience the benefits of robust and healthy digestion.

—MEREDITH

67

Millions of people suffer from irregular bowel patterns. Feeling backed up is not fun, and the consequences of constipation can be wide ranging, from hemorrhoids to general discomfort and even toxin reabsorption, which may cause fatigue, headaches, or cold-like symptoms.

Modern lifestyle factors can contribute to constipation, including—you guessed it!—not eating enough fiber, lack of hydration, a sedentary lifestyle, changes in your routine, discomfort or shame around going in public, and stress or other mental health issues. Do any of these sound familiar? You're not alone. The good news? Regular stool is all about routine, and by establishing a consistent poop routine, you can help train your body to eliminate at the same time each day. For most people, the time of day is in the morning, but that's not necessarily the case for everyone.

These are our top tips for establishing a regular elimination routine:

→ **EAT REGULAR MEALS**
Eating at regular intervals is the number-one way to bring about healthy bowel habits. If your eating schedule is erratic, your digestive rhythm can disappear. We recommend trying to eat each of your meals around the same time each day, with three to four hours in between. Snacking should be limited because it can disrupt the digestive process.

→ **IF YOU HAVE TO GO—GO!**
Don't ignore the urge to have a bowel movement. Delaying elimination can lead to constipation, irregularity, and extreme discomfort.

→ **INCREASE FIBER INTAKE**
Gradually increasing your fiber intake helps bulk up stools and promote regularity.

→ **STAY HYDRATED**
Hydration is a huge factor in regularity. When the colon is hydrated, it helps us to eliminate swiftly and smoothly. Dehydration can cause constipation because the body retains water instead of releasing it into the colon, leading to dry, hard stools that are difficult to pass. Stay hydrated by drinking plenty of water and consuming water-rich foods. More on this in Chapter 4: Help Your Self Hydrate (page 118).

→ **MOVE YOUR BODY**
Physical activity helps manage stress and promotes healthy colon contractions. Move your body to move your bowels.

→ **CONSIDER PROBIOTICS**
Probiotics can help balance gut bacteria, which may improve bowel regularity. Foods like yogurt, kefir, and fermented vegetables are good probiotic sources.

→ **MANAGE STRESS**
Gut health is connected to brain health, and vice versa. Managing stress levels can help improve the quality of your digestion. Stress hormones activate the "fight or flight" response, which can divert blood flow away from the digestive system and slow down the digestive process.

Check Your Chart

We're not talking astrology here. We want to introduce you to a resource that's going to become your best friend when it comes to healthy, regular elimination: the Bristol Stool Chart. Whenever you poop, compare what you see to the chart. A 1 or 2 means you could use some hydration from water and eat more water-rich foods. It could also mean you've overeaten foods that are too dry or salty. A 3 or 4 means you're in good shape, and a 5, 6, or 7 could be caused by many issues that indicate an upset stomach, from food intolerances to infection. The range can be mild to severe.

BRISTOL STOOL CHART

CONSTIPATION		
		1. Hard, separate pellet-like lumps that are difficult to pass
		2. Lumpy, sausage-shaped stool

NORMAL		
		3. Sausage-shaped stool with cracks on the surface
		4. Sausage-shaped stool but smooth and soft (like a snake)

DIARRHEA		
		5. Blobs that are soft and pass easily
		6. Mushy stool in the form of fluffy pieces with ragged edges
		7. Entirely liquid; no solid pieces

Bloating 101

Abdominal bloating is a widespread symptom that affects people of all ages, and it's no fun.

Its underlying causes are not fully understood but may be related to factors including gut hypersensitivity, compromised microbiota, and abnormal abdominal reflexes (translation: a reduced ability to handle gas). While there is medication to ease symptoms of gas and bloating, we recommend trying to address it holistically first through diet and lifestyle.

As discussed on page 62, the gut microbiome and the migrating motor complex (MMC) are major factors in regulating symptoms of gas and bloating—with resting digestion being imperative—but it's not everything. Food combining, eating habits and cadence, gulping, and drinking too much water with food (diluting gastric juices) are all potential factors in increasing your chances of getting gas.

Here are some common reasons for bloating, and what you can do about them:

Slow Bowel Movements
It goes without saying, but if you are prone to constipation, your chances of suffering from bloating will be much higher. When stool builds up in the colon, it can naturally cause gas and bloating. We've already touched on many important factors to address and improve bowel function—microbiome health, resting digestion, and good hydration are all important in improving the process of elimination. Of course, there are times when the bowels move more slowly (e.g., when traveling). If it isn't chronic, our best advice is to not stress or think about it too much. This is normal and nothing to be concerned about.

Hormonal Changes
Many people who menstruate experience bloating before and during their menstrual periods, or during menopause, due to hormonal fluctuations, particularly an increase in progesterone. If this is the case for you, go easy on your digestive system during this time. Skip the seven-course dinner and go for something fiber rich and hydrating.

Irritable Bowel Syndrome (IBS)
This is a common disorder that affects the large intestine, causing symptoms such as bloating, gas, abdominal pain, and changes in bowel habits. IBS is not a single-symptom diagnosis but a more generalized condition and can vary widely among individuals.

Celiac Disease
This is an autoimmune disorder where the ingestion of gluten leads to damage in the small intestine, resulting in bloating and other digestive issues. While celiac disease is diagnosable, there is a spectrum of gluten sensitivity. We recommend paying attention to these foods and noting whether they leave you bloated.

Too Much Fiber?
If you are new to a plant-based diet, consuming large amounts of fiber-rich foods like beans, lentils, broccoli, and whole grains can cause gas and bloating. So, if you are just starting out on this path, we recommend gradually increasing your fiber intake to help your digestive system adjust. You will also want to make sure that you are eating diverse fiber sources, which will improve the quality of your gut bacteria and reduce the chances of gas or bloating with fiber intake.

Carbonated Drinks
We know this is a hard one to hear if you love bubble water. But consuming fizzy drinks can introduce excess gas into the digestive system, leading to bloating. With that said, if you have a healthy gut, you will not necessarily be gassy after drinking carbonated drinks. Common sense measures like not drinking too quickly and mostly consuming them separate from food are important. Pay attention to your body; if carbonated drinks negatively impact your digestive system, we recommend limiting them.

Dairy Products
Many people suffer from lactose intolerance, which can easily cause bloating, gas, and discomfort. While we aren't addressing dairy in this book in depth, it should be noted that many people are lactose intolerant. Genetics play a role in this, and if you think it is an issue for you, again, pay attention.

Swallowing Air (Aerophagia)
Yes, this can cause bloating, but it is primarily a lifestyle consideration, as it includes eating too fast, talking with food in your mouth, chewing gum, and drinking through straws.

Food Combining

While we don't buy into elaborate food combining, we do believe in following this simple rule to aid digestion: Eat water-rich foods before heavy, dry, or protein-rich foods.

The practice of strategically eating foods together or separately to improve nutrient absorption is a big topic of conversation in the food and health world. There are some extravagant claims and complicated theories out there, none of which are backed by science, so we stay away from them. It is worth noting, however, that food combining has long been practiced in many cultures outside of the US. Many Middle Eastern food traditions, as well as Jewish dietary laws mandating the separation of meat and dairy, exist as rituals of purity and proper digestion.

We have found that eating water-rich foods like melons, grapes, or cucumber after a heavy meal causes gas and bloating, because they move through the digestive system quickly and can get backed up against those heavier foods. The exception to this rule is if a water-rich food is fermented (like pickles versus cucumbers), as fermented foods tend to digest more slowly and combine well with other foods. Which brings us to . . .

Fermented Foods

We love fermented foods for so many reasons: They support our microbiome, improve digestion, and boost nutrient absorption, to name a few. Decades ago, we used to eat more fermented foods as a culture in the form of pickles, traditionally fermented sourdough breads, and dairy, such as milk and yogurt. But with the industrialization of our food supply, and the advent of refrigeration and pasteurization, fermentation has gone by the wayside. Before pasteurization, fermentation was the primary method for food preservation. We relied on the fermentation process to preserve fruits and vegetables, and it was a significant source of support for the microbiome and gut microbial diversity. Other cultures, notably Asian cultures, still consume a significant number of fermented foods and experience better health because of it.

Fermented foods are important because they are packed with gut-healthy probiotics. By supporting good gut bacteria, they also enhance nutrient absorption, help regulate bowel movements, and boost the immune system. Oh, and they taste good! Adding fermented foods and condiments is a great way to add satisfying umami flavor and boost to almost any dish.

Our favorite ferments are:

- SAUERKRAUT

- KIMCHEE

- PICKLES FERMENTED IN BRINE

- TEMPEH

- NATTO

- TRADITIONALLY FERMENTED BREADS (E.G., NATURAL SOURDOUGH)

"If I could name one thing I've consistently done over the years that has made the most positive impact on my gut health, it would be focusing on eating fermented foods—primarily sauerkraut. Once I developed a taste for kraut (which was always kind of there), I started to add it to everything—salads, sandwiches, pasta, etc. The flavor is quite umami and adds a nice salty brine to many things. I love it. The most interesting part of getting my gut health in check has been that my sweet tooth is virtually non-existent these days and I'm happily very regular."

—MEREDITH

INGESTIBLES

Prebiotics

Prebiotics are food components that our bodies can't digest but that support the growth of beneficial bacteria in our gut.[15] Prebiotics are typically complex carbohydrates, including fructans and galactans, and because we can't digest them, they arrive largely intact in the colon, serving as nutrients for beneficial bacteria.[16]

Prebiotics can be taken in supplemental form,[17] but they can also be found in many food sources. Although we do need prebiotics for a healthy digestive system, overeating, or eating large quantities of prebiotic foods, can cause digestive issues, especially in people with sensitive digestion. All prebiotic foods contain inulin, a type of soluble fiber and prebiotic found in many plants. It resists digestion in the small intestine and ferments in the colon, where it feeds beneficial gut bacteria.

Foods that are naturally high in inulin and rich in prebiotics include:

- APPLES
- ASPARAGUS
- BARLEY
- CHICORY ROOT
- DANDELION GREENS
- GARLIC
- JERUSALEM ARTICHOKE
- KONJAC ROOT
- ONIONS AND LEEKS
- OATS
- SEAWEED

Probiotics

The word "probiotic" has started to pop up everywhere, often without meaning (on cereals and other processed foods). Probiotics are live bacteria and yeasts that have beneficial effects on the body, and particularly on gut health. Many fermented foods naturally contain probiotics, and eating these foods is the best way to consume them.

However, if you feel like you need an extra boost, there are also high-quality probiotic supplements available. We recommend seeking brands that are third-party tested, high CFU (colony-forming units) products with diverse strains, and, ideally, strains backed by clinical research for specific health benefits. To effectively increase probiotic intake, we prefer relying on fermented foods and smartly supplementing with products that adhere to quality standards.

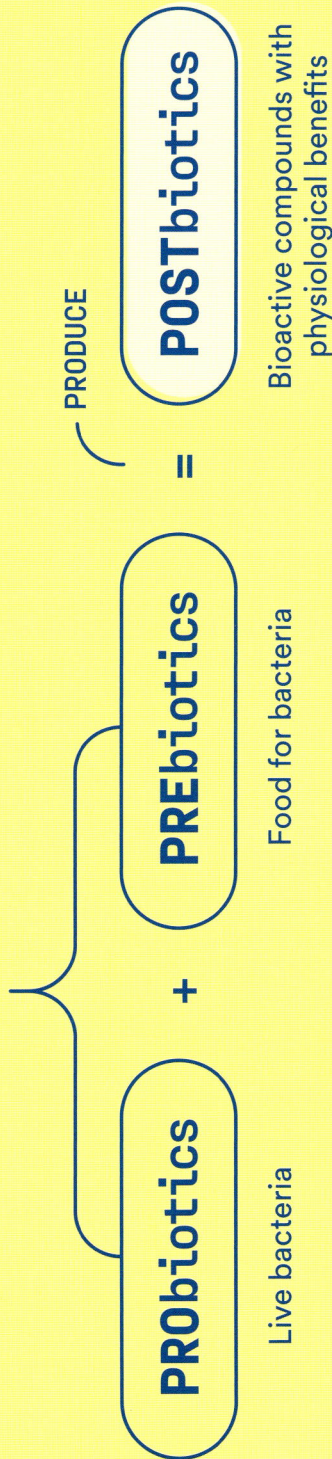

POSTbiotics

Bioactive compounds with physiological benefits

PRODUCE

=

PREbiotics

Food for bacteria

+

SYNbiotics

PRObiotics

Live bacteria

Postbiotics

Postbiotics are byproducts of digestion, and like probiotics and prebiotics, they are believed to contribute to gut health. Postbiotics include microbial metabolites, such as short-chain fatty acids,[18] enzymes, bacterial lysates, cell wall components, vitamins, amino acids, and peptides. Unlike live probiotics, postbiotics are nonliving components that can enhance health by supporting immune function, reducing inflammation, improving gut barrier integrity, promoting the growth of beneficial gut bacteria, and aiding in nutrient absorption.

Postbiotics are found naturally in fermented foods or are available as supplements. They offer a promising avenue for enhancing gut health and overall well-being without the need to consume live bacteria. Food sources of probiotics and postbiotics:

● FERMENTED CHEESE (DAIRY AND NONDAIRY)
Cheese that contains postbiotics from its fermentation process.

● KEFIR
A fermented milk drink with a diverse microbial community that generates postbiotics.

● KIMCHI
A traditional Korean side dish of fermented vegetables that produce pre-, pro-, and postbiotics through the fermentation process.

● KOMBUCHA
A fermented tea beverage produced by bacteria and yeast.

● MISO
Our favorite Japanese seasoning made from fermented soybeans.

● NATTO
Fermented soybeans that are a rich source of unique postbiotics.

● PICKLES
Cucumbers or other vegetables fermented in brine.

● SAUERKRAUT
Raw cabbage that has been fermented and produces pre-, pro-, and postbiotics from the activity of Lactobacillus bacteria.

● TEMPEH
A fermented soybean product that contains various postbiotics.

● YOGURT (DAIRY AND NONDAIRY)
Contains live cultures that produce postbiotics like short-chain fatty acids during fermentation.

73

"

My digestion has become so regular that I go to the bathroom at the same exact time every morning, and instead of sitting on the toilet for hours, I'm in and out in just a few minutes. This wasn't always the case for me.

I love good probiotics and supplements, but for a while I wasn't eating enough fiber. Once I started eating fiber-rich foods like sweet potatoes, lots of steamed vegetables, and whole grains regularly throughout the day, my digestion did a one-eighty. When I am especially good about my fiber intake, I can see a difference in my stool quality the next day.

—KAT

● **7:00**^{AM}

Upon waking, I drink one to two glasses of room-temperature water. If my digestion is feeling off, I add a tablespoon of apple cider vinegar (ACV) to kickstart things.

In its raw and unfiltered form, ACV contains a small amount of probiotics and may help stimulate the production of stomach acid.

● **7:30**^{AM}

Water usually gets my digestive system going, and I poop quickly. The shape and texture of my stool will indicate to me what I need to be consuming throughout the day—whether I need more water or more fiber. (See the Bristol Stool Chart on page 69 for details on what your poop means.)

● **8:00**^{AM}

I make an Americano with organic espresso, adding some alkaline water to ensure I'm not starting the day too acidic.

● **10:30**^{AM} (BREAKFAST)

I have breakfast, which is usually a smoothie that's rich in fiber, protein, and prebiotics. I don't add fruit, but load it up with frozen avocados, greens, cauliflower, protein, and nut butter.

I practice 16:8 intermittent fasting, meaning that I fast for sixteen hours and eat within an eight-hour window. I've experienced great benefits from it personally, including better focus.

● **12:00**^{PM}

To stay hydrated, I drink a big glass of warm water with lemon. I sometimes go crazy and add electrolytes. I never drink cold water, as it can slow digestion by constricting blood vessels and irritate the nerves in your stomach. Room- (or body-) temperature water is easier on digestion.

● **1:00**^{PM} (LUNCH)

I'll have a lunch that is rich in protein and fermented foods. My mom is a macrobiotic chef, so I've been eating fermented foods since I was a baby.

I keep a stash of fermented foods I've made in the fridge, and I have a little something that's fermented (sauerkraut!) ahead of every meal. For lunch, I opt for a macro bowl with tempeh, tofu, or beans as my protein source.

● **3:00**^{PM}

I eat my poop muffin. This recipe is so rich in fiber—it keeps me full until dinner and helps my digestion run smoothly the next day. (See the recipe on page 81.)

● **6:30**^{PM} (DINNER)

My last meal ends, which means that I start eating dinner around 5:45 to 6 p.m. Soups and stews are where it's at for dinner—they help you ease into resting your digestive system. I almost always load up on steamed veggies at dinnertime too.

Trust me, if you want to see your stool log, you will want to incorporate a bunch of steamed veggies and complex carbs like sweet potatoes into your dinner. Skip the raw foods at night.

● **8:00**^{PM}

I take my Ritual Synbiotic+, which is our 3-in-1 product that contains pre-, pro-, and postbiotics. I take most of my supplements before bed, except for my stress adaptogens (because I need those stress-adaptive benefits during the day).

75

● **6:30**AM

I wake up and drink a big glass of room-temperature filtered water—usually about 16 to 20 ounces. I used to add lemon to it, but I've stopped craving it and now prefer the water au naturale.

● **7:00**AM

One of my favorite parts of the day is my morning Americano. I drink it black or with a splash of nut milk. If I haven't pooped by now, this is always when it will happen.

● **8:00**AM

If it's cold outside I'll drink some warm water or herbal tea to get me out the door for a walk or a workout after school drop-off. If I feel hungry, I'll have a piece of fruit. I try to hydrate and eliminate before I eat anything substantial.

● **10–10:30**AM (BREAKFAST)

Sometimes I eat earlier than this, and some-times later. I honestly don't like breakfast food or smoothies all that much, so breakfast always con-fuses me. On the day of writing this, I had a left-over tempeh dish from the night before. Many of my breakfasts are leftovers.

● **1:00**PM (LUNCH)

I always eat a big salad or bowl of some sort with beans, grains, seeds, avocado, and something fer-mented, drizzled with olive oil or tahini dressing. Sometimes it also includes leftovers from the night before. I love a good dipping sauce to keep things interesting.

● **2:30**PM

Lots of tea and maybe a little sweet, like chocolate. I love jasmine tea and will often poop after lunch if I have it.

● **5:00**PM

I always have a transitional beverage to ease into the evening and get me in the mood for making dinner and being present for that time of day. I'll drink wine occasionally, but more and more it's a nonalcoholic beverage with herbs like L-theanine, an amino acid primarily found in tea leaves, known for its calming effects (discussed in Chapter 6: Help Your Self Stress Less, page 168). It is found primarily in green tea and in certain types of mushrooms. I've found it to be highly effective for winding down.

● **6–6:30**PM (DINNER)

I don't spend a ton of time making dinner but gen-erally enjoy the process. We do veggie tacos, pasta with lots of fresh herbs and beans, grain bowls—things of that nature are always in rotation. Some of my favorite meals happen when I am limited to the random ingredients we have in the fridge.

● **8:00**PM (WIND DOWN)

After my daughter goes to bed, I've gotten into a nice routine of deep stretching after applying my skin care. I can't begin to describe how good it feels. I'll use an ice roller on my face to help stretch and diffuse essential oils.

I try to switch it up depending on what the evening looks like, but my goal is always to deeply relax before I climb into bed. I often take a mag-nesium citrate supplement at night to help with digestion the next morning.

● **9:00**PM

I can't say that I recommend it if you have sleep issues, but my husband and I love to watch a movie or show before bed. We try not to scroll or be on our phones and limit ourselves to only watching something we're both enjoying. I do mix it up with reading quite a bit. I know blue light before bed isn't great, but we're all doing the best we can!

We know that the topic of digestive health doesn't always feel like cocktail party conversation.

However, we want to shatter the taboos that surround discussing gut health. We hope that the information in this chapter helps you feel more open to having the conversation and considering how digestive health plays a central role in your overall well-being, significantly influencing how you age, sleep, manage energy, cope with stress, and even experience sexual health.

Now that we've explored the importance of nurturing our digestive health, it's time to put that knowledge into action with some delicious, gut-friendly recipes. After all, you can't enjoy food if you're experiencing digestive discomfort.

The following pages are filled with meals that not only taste amazing but also work to support your digestion. The recipes are packed with fiber, prebiotics, probiotics—all the good things—and soothing ingredients to keep your gut happy and balanced.

The Recipes

→ Kat's "Poop Muffins"

→ Super Seedy Flax Crackers

→ Warm Kale Salad with Tahini and Buckwheat Crispies

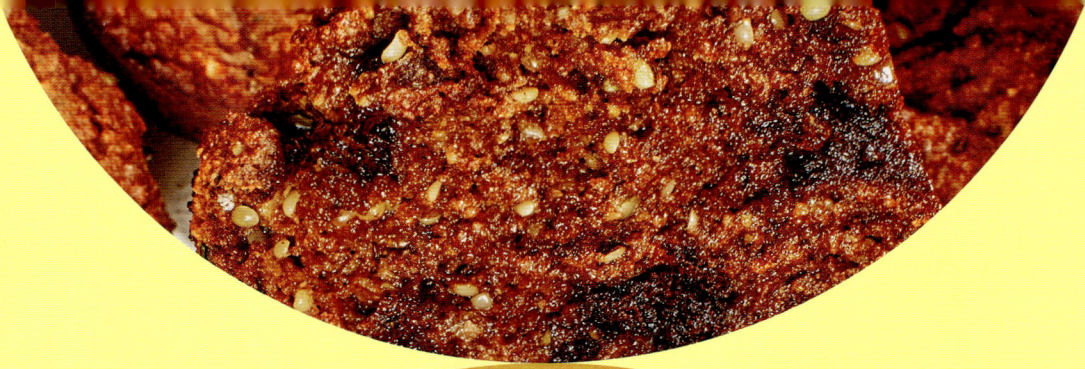

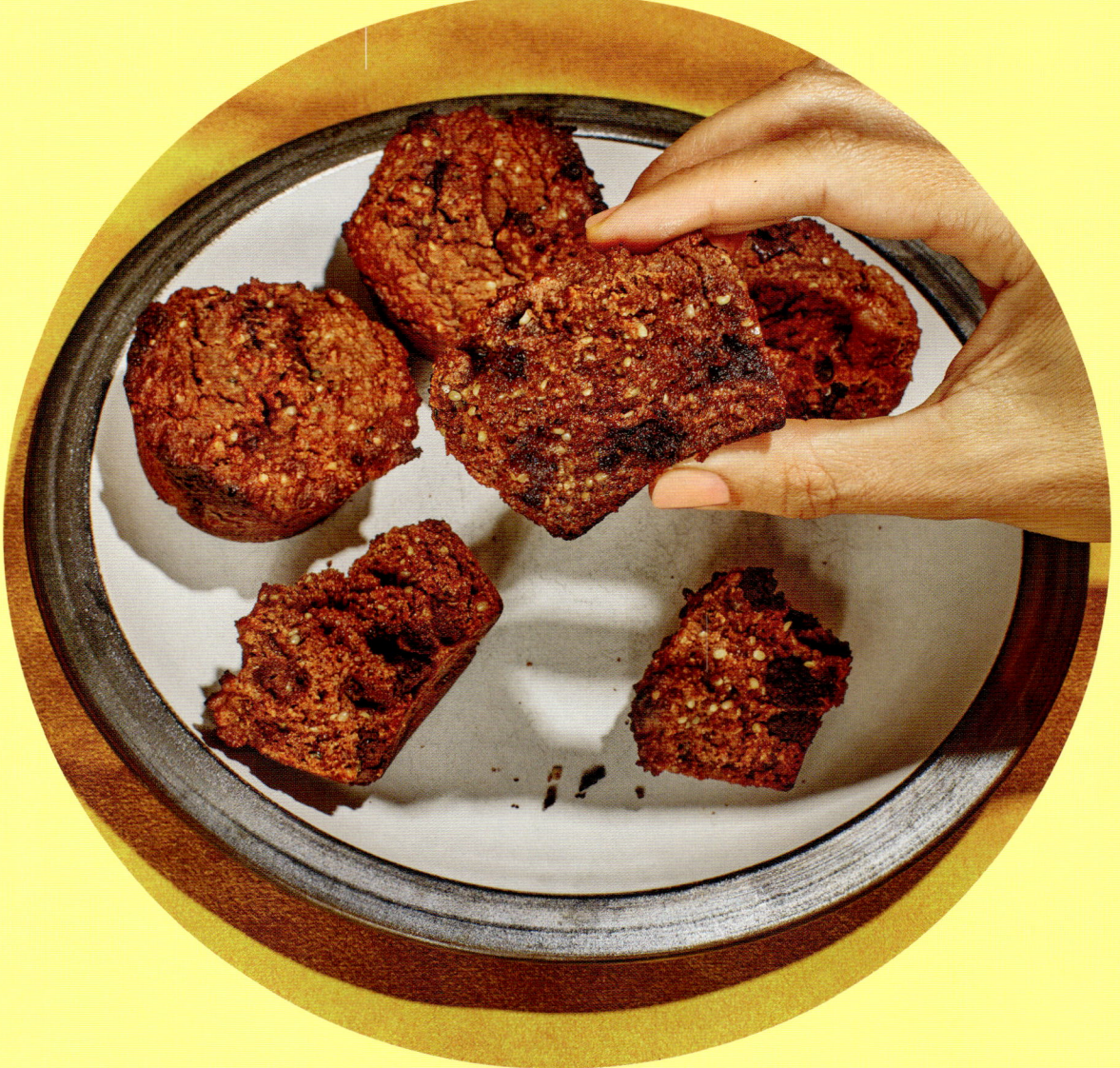

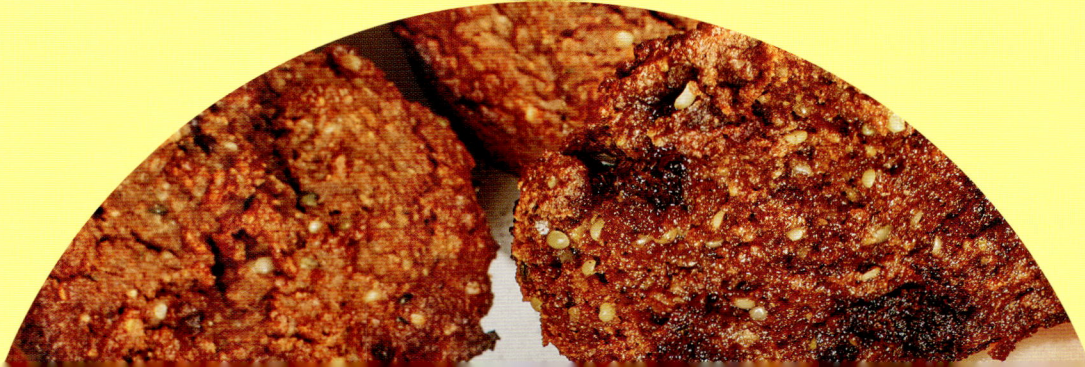

Kat's "Poop Muffins"

These muffins are the perfect high-protein breakfast snack and are guaranteed to get your digestive system moving in all the right ways. Kat swears by them.

If you aren't familiar with allulose, it is a low-calorie sweetener that has minimal impact on blood sugar. It naturally occurs in small amounts in certain fruits and foods like wheat, figs, and raisins. If you aren't concerned with sugar, you can substitute coconut sugar in this recipe.

MAKES ABOUT 12 STANDARD-SIZE MUFFINS

2 tablespoons ground flaxseed

1½ cups (140 g) Bob's Red Mill Paleo baking flour (or other paleo flour mix)

1 teaspoon baking soda

2 tablespoons cocoa powder

2 tablespoons hemp seeds

2 tablespoons chia seeds, ground

¼ cup (50 g) allulose or coconut sugar

Pinch of salt

½ cup (120 ml) non-dairy milk of your choice

¼ cup (60 ml) melted coconut oil

1 tablespoon apple cider vinegar

1 teaspoon vanilla extract

⅓ cup (60 g) 100% dark chocolate chips

How to make?

→ Preheat

Preheat your oven to 350°F (175°C) and line a muffin pan with paper liners or grease with coconut oil.

→ Prepare the flax egg

In a small bowl, mix the ground flaxseed with 5 tablespoons of water. Let it sit for 5 to 10 minutes until it forms a gel-like consistency.

→ Mix dry ingredients

In a large bowl, whisk together the paleo flour, baking soda, cocoa powder, hemp seeds, chia seeds, allulose, and a pinch of salt.

→ Combine wet ingredients

In another bowl, whisk together the flax egg, nut milk, melted coconut oil, apple cider vinegar, and vanilla extract until well combined.

→ Mix wet and dry ingredients

Pour the wet ingredients into the dry ingredients and stir until just combined. Be careful not to overmix. Gently fold in the chocolate chips.

→ Scoop the batter

Divide the batter evenly among the muffin cups, filling each about two-thirds full.

→ Bake

Place the muffin pan in the preheated oven and bake for 18 to 22 minutes, or until a toothpick inserted in the center of a muffin comes out clean.

→ Cool

Allow the muffins to cool in the pan for 5 minutes, then transfer to a wire rack to cool completely.

→ Serve

These muffins are best enjoyed slightly warm, allowing the chocolate chips to melt a bit inside. Store any leftovers in an airtight container at room temperature for up to 3 days.

81

Super Seedy
Flax Crackers

**MAKES ABOUT
3 DOZEN CRACKERS**

2 cups (330 g) flax seeds

½ cup (80 g) chia seeds

½ cup (75 g) sesame seeds

½ cup (70 g) hulled
sunflower seeds

½ cup (65 g) hulled pumpkin
seeds

½ cup (60 g) hemp seeds
(optional)

¼ cup (30 g) nutritional
yeast (optional)

2 tablespoons turmeric
powder

1 teaspoon salt

1 teaspoon garlic powder

1 teaspoon onion powder

1 teaspoon ground cumin

2 cups (480 ml) water (may
need a little more to spread)

1 to 2 tablespoons olive oil
(optional, for moisture)

How to make?

Preheat the oven to 350°F (175°C). (If you prefer to make the crackers in a dehydrator, see below.)

In a medium bowl, mix the flax, chia, sesame, pumpkin, and hemp seeds (if using) and the optional nutritional yeast with the turmeric, salt, garlic powder, onion powder, and cumin. Add 2 cups (480 ml) water and stir well to combine. Allow the mixture to sit for about 30 minutes to let the water absorb and the batter to thicken. The flax and chia seeds together will create a gel-like consistency, and the batter should be easy to spread without being runny. If it feels too thick to spread, you can stir in ½ cup (120 ml) more water, or more if needed. Once the batter has a good consistency, stir in the olive oil, if using.

Using an offset spatula, spread the batter onto a parchment-lined baking sheet in a thin, even layer (about ⅛ inch/3 mm thick). Using a sharp knife, score the batter into 2-inch (5 cm) squares to create about 36 crackers in all.

Bake in the preheated oven for 25 to 30 minutes, or until the edges are golden brown and the sheet of crackers feels dry and firm to the touch. It will naturally separate from the parchment paper.

Remove from the oven and allow the crackers to cool. They will continue to firm up as they cool. Once cool, break them apart at the scored lines. Crackers can be stored for about 1 month in a tightly sealed container.

→ Dehydrator Option

While baking in the oven yields great results, we prefer to make these crackers in a dehydrator, which achieves extra crispiness without the risk of burning them.

Make the batter as described above. Preheat the dehydrator to 120°F (50°C). When it's time to spread the batter on the baking sheet, spread it on dehydrator trays instead and dehydrate at 120°F (50°C) for up to 12 hours or overnight. Check to make sure the crackers are completely dry before removing them from the trays; you may need to flip them and dehydrate for an extra hour or two.

"Extremely high in fiber, so much better for you than store-bought crackers, and surprisingly simple to make—these are a triple win. I make these on a monthly basis, and if I double the batch, they will last for close to two months.

Once you get the hang of the process, you can play around with different seeds or eliminate the ones you don't have on hand—the only nonnegotiables are the flax and chia seeds. My favorite version includes nutritional yeast for an added cheesy flavor."

—MEREDITH

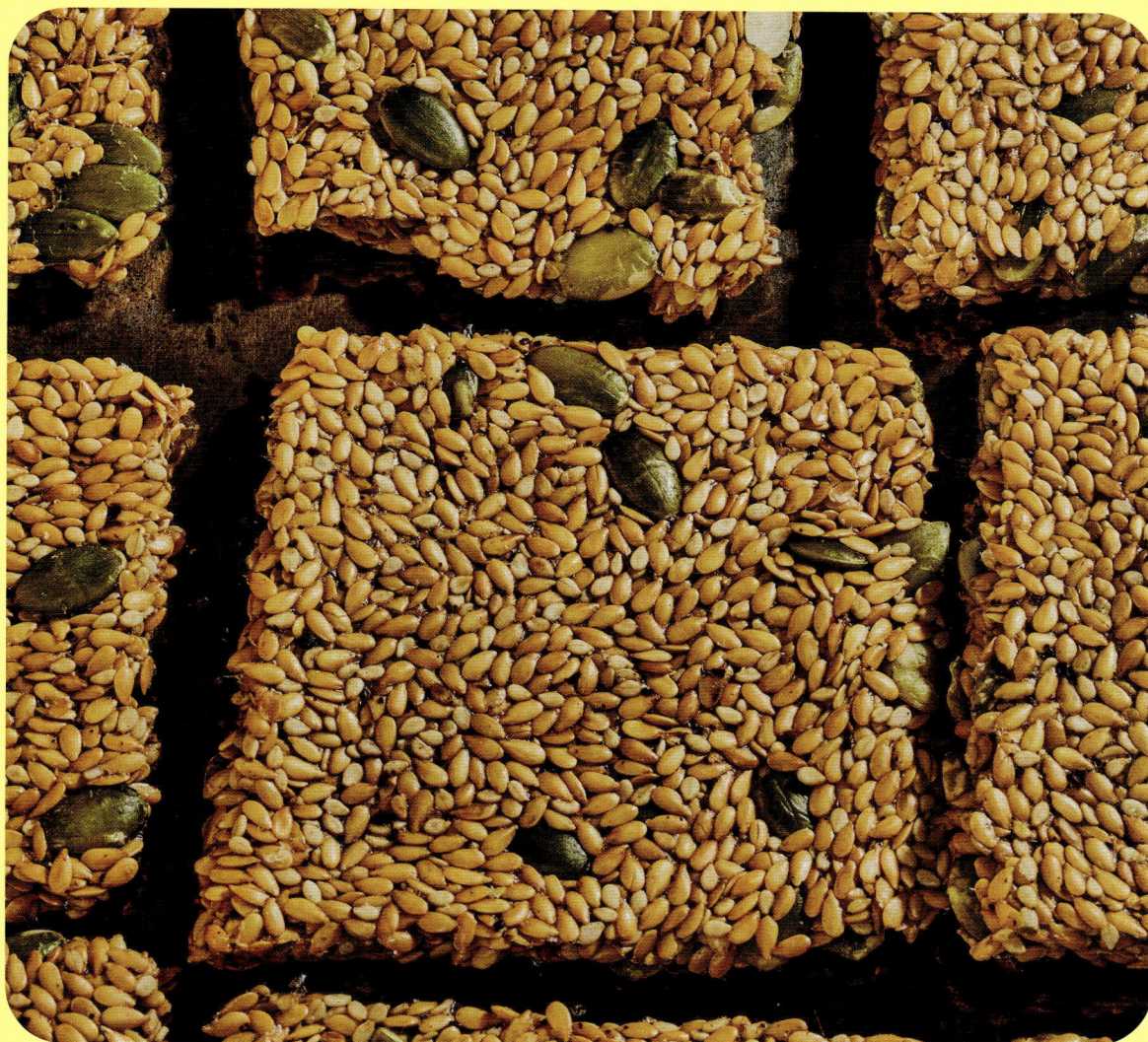

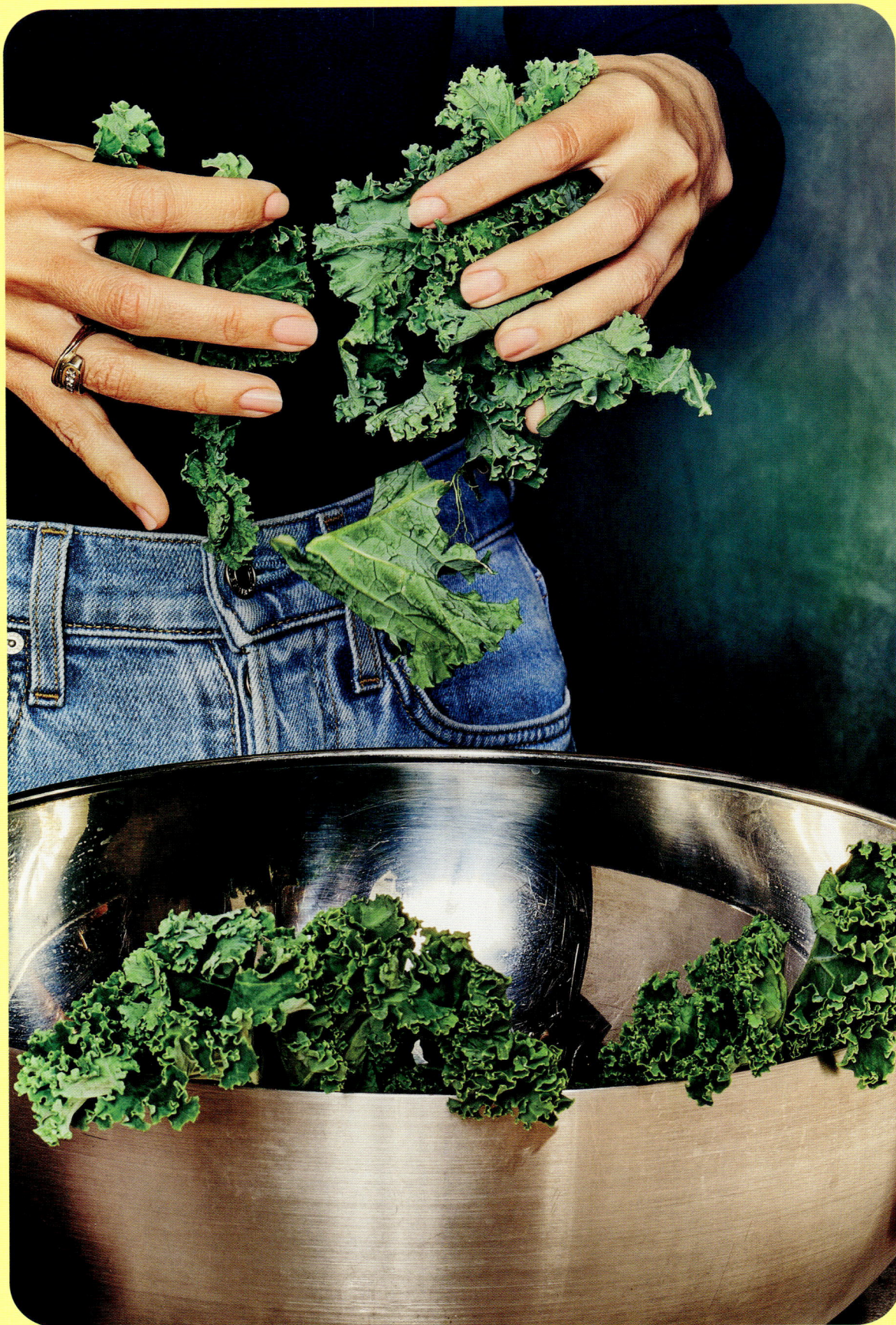

Warm Kale Salad with Tahini and Buckwheat Crispies

Kale will never be overrated, in our opinion.
It's hearty and holds up under any dressing.

MAKES ENOUGH FOR
4 PEOPLE

FOR THE KALE:

2 large bunches kale

2 tablespoons olive oil

1 teaspoon sea salt

FOR THE DRESSING:

½ cup (120 ml) tahini

Juice of 1 lemon

1 clove garlic, minced

2 green onions, finely chopped

1 handful fresh parsley leaves

1 handful fresh cilantro leaves

FOR THE BUCKWHEAT CRISPIES:

1 cup (175 g) buckwheat groats

2 tablespoons olive oil

2 teaspoons sea salt

How to make?

→ Soak

Soak the buckwheat groats for 20 to 30 minutes while you prepare the other ingredients. This helps with the cooking time.

→ Prepare the kale

Preheat the oven to warm (170°F to 200°F / 75°C to 95°C). Rinse the kale and cut off about 1 inch (2.5 cm) of the stem to separate the leaves. (No need to remove the remaining stems.)

Dry the kale with towels, place in a single layer on one or two parchment-lined baking sheets, and toss with the olive oil and sea salt to coat.

Roast the kale in the warm oven for 8 to 10 minutes. This will soften the stems and make the leaves crisp.

→ While the kale roasts, make the dressing

Using a whisk or an immersion blender, mix the tahini, 1 cup (240 ml) water, the lemon juice, garlic, green onions, parsley, and cilantro until smooth. The dressing can be stored in an airtight container in the refrigerator for up to 4 days.

→ Make the buckwheat crispies

Drain the buckwheat. Turn the oven temperature up to 350°F (175°C) and preheat. Line a baking sheet with parchment paper. Toss the buckwheat with the olive oil and sea salt and spread it on the lined baking sheet. Roast for 15 to 20 minutes, stirring every 5 minutes to ensure the buckwheat cooks evenly.

→ Arrange

Arrange the kale on a serving platter or individual serving plates. Drizzle the greens with the tahini dressing, garnish with the buckwheat crispies, and serve immediately.

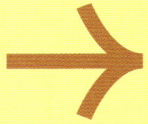
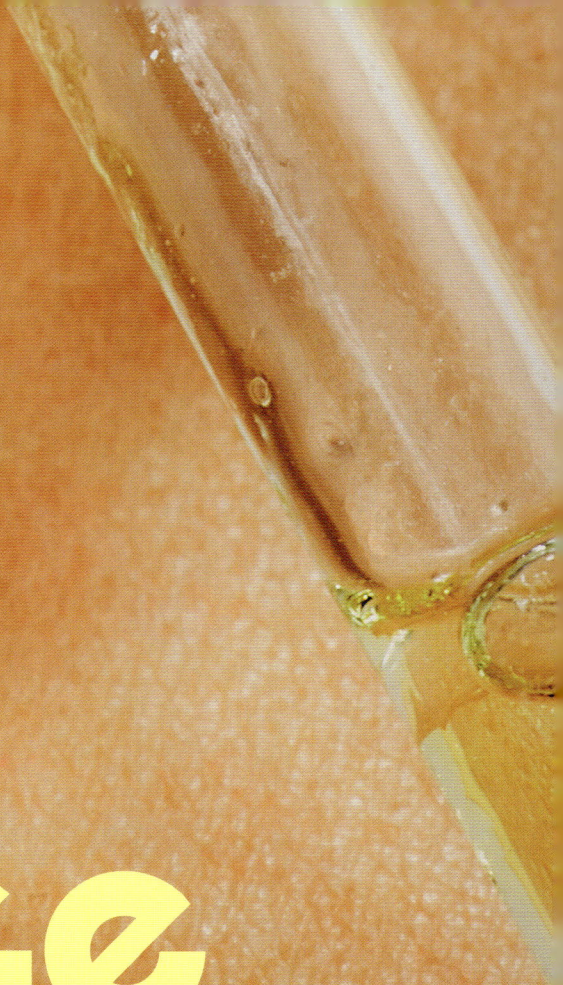

Age

Well

"

When I was in my mid-twenties, after years of "healthy eating" (or so I thought), I started to develop skin issues—severely dry patches, eczema-like spots, and dry scalp. I was devastated because I was sure I'd been doing everything right. I was living in NYC at the time, and I went to a top dermatologist who diagnosed me with psoriasis. I left that appointment with all kinds of prescriptions and foams, but I knew that going on meds wasn't going to be the answer for me long-term. So, I stepped back and tried to evaluate everything that could have triggered this reaction—from foods and topicals to environmental factors.

What I discovered was that although my diet was pretty good, I possibly wasn't getting enough healthy fats, and my skin care products weren't truly effective enough to combat cold NYC winters. I also had a high-intensity job and unmanaged stress that was causing flare-ups. So, I decided to take matters into my own hands. I began experimenting with healing, plant-based skin care ingredients, which would ultimately lead to the creation of my skin care line, Nucifera. Ultimately, it was the combination of internal changes (my diet) and external changes (skin care products and lifestyle factors) that made a positive impact.

Now, almost twenty years later, I feel that I can see the benefits of truly nourishing and hydrating my skin and the longer-term impact that had on my skin's tone, texture, and quality. I almost feel grateful for the skin issues I had in my twenties, because they forced me to care for my skin.

88

I truly believe that our skin is a window into how we care for ourselves. Everyone's skin is unique and reactive in different ways, but the foundations of good food, healthy relationships, and quality skin care products can work for everyone.
—MEREDITH

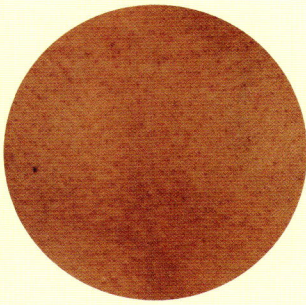

The taboos around aging are wide-ranging and can often be so negatively charged. We should all want to age! Otherwise, what is the alternative? We are not here to tell you that it should be your goal to prevent aging, or that this is even possible. The reality is that we all age, our skin ages, and this is a natural (healthy) and highly desirable process.

While our skin does serve as a window into our broader health—revealing stress, inflammation, nutrient deficiencies, or dehydration—it's essential not to become overly fixated on appearance. Aging well is about supporting our skin's resilience, vibrance, and radiance over time, rather than simply trying to erase lines or imperfections. True wellness embraces the balance of caring for our skin as part of a holistic approach to health. Radiant skin isn't just about what you apply on the surface; it's deeply connected to our nourishment and daily habits.

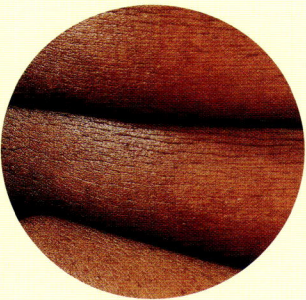

The Basics

Why our skin ages

Skin aging is a complex process influenced by intrinsic (genetic) and extrinsic (external/environmental) factors. Studies suggest that genetics may account for approximately 60 percent of the variation in skin aging, with epigenetic or environmental factors like sun exposure, diet, and lifestyle making up the remaining 40 percent.[1]

The good news here is that even if we weren't born with naturally flawless skin, we do have a lot of influence over the health of our skin through lifestyle choices and increasingly effective skin care technologies.

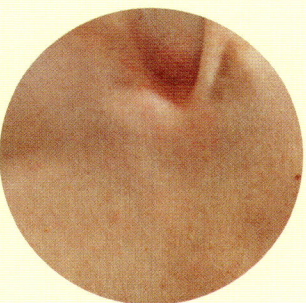

Intrinsic Aging

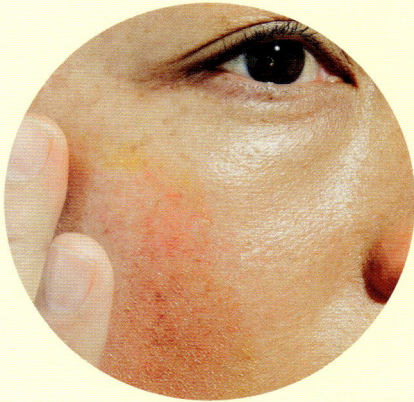

Intrinsic aging, also known as chronological aging, is the skin's natural aging process that occurs over time. This type of aging is largely (although not entirely) determined by our genetic makeup and includes cellular aging, hormonal aging, and slowing skin cell turnover. Intrinsic skin aging is also influenced by hormonal changes that occur with age, including the decreased production of sex hormones like estrogen and progesterone associated with menopause. For men, the dip in testosterone is the primary cause of increased signs of intrinsic aging.

Below are the skin-aging factors that are mostly determined by genetics, which contribute to intrinsic aging:

COLLAGEN PRODUCTION

Collagen is a protein our bodies produce that helps maintain our skin's shape, moisture, and elasticity. As we age, the genes that are responsible for producing collagen become less active, leading to wrinkles, fine lines, skin sagging, and thinning. Estrogen promotes the production of collagen, and as estrogen levels decline in perimenopause and menopause, collagen production will decline as well.

ELASTIN PRODUCTION

Like collagen, elastin is a protein that gives elasticity and flexibility to the tissues in the body. Genetic factors determine elastin production and decline with age, leading to the loss of skin elasticity.

DNA REPAIR MECHANISMS

Genetics play a crucial role in the rate of DNA repair mechanisms, and this function decreases with age. DNA repair is crucial for maintaining skin stability and preventing mutations. DNA damage may lead to cellular dysfunction and visible signs of aging.

UV-INDUCED DAMAGE

Our genes also determine how susceptible we are to UV radiation from the sun's rays. UV radiation damages our skin through photoaging, which is the premature aging of our skin that shows up as wrinkles, irregular pigmentation, dryness, skin roughness, and early signs of skin cancer.[2]

REACTIVE OXYGEN SPECIES (ROS)

You may have heard the term "ROS" being tossed around in skin care discussions. ROS are molecules produced in the skin when oxygen is exposed to environmental factors like pollution, UV rays, and visible light, and these molecules can cause skin aging, skin diseases including cancer, and UV-induced photodamage of the skin.[3]

ANTIOXIDANT ENZYMES

These are proteins, which are regulated by our genes and are part of the body's antioxidant defense system, preventing or slowing cell damage caused by free radicals (unstable molecules that the body produces as a reaction to environmental factors). These free radicals cause what is called oxidative stress, which can cause inflammation and damage the skin.

TELOMERE LENGTH

Telomeres are structures made from DNA sequences and proteins that "cap" the ends of our chromosomes, preventing them from becoming frayed. Telomere length shortens with age, and as this happens, cells lose their ability to divide and function properly, resulting in signs of aging such as wrinkles, loss of elasticity, and slower wound healing. The length of telomeres and the rate of their shortening is largely determined by genetic factors.[4]

Extrinsic Aging

Environmental factors and lifestyle choices contribute to extrinsic aging. Some of the most common factors that cause extrinsic aging include:

SUN EXPOSURE

UV radiation from the sun is the primary cause of photoaging. UV rays can damage the DNA in skin cells, break down collagen, and lead to the formation of free radicals, which accelerate aging. We'll discuss this more later in the chapter.

SMOKING

We've all heard it, and it should go without saying, but tobacco smoke wreaks havoc on the skin. It contains toxins that damage collagen and elastin, leading to premature wrinkles and sagging.

POLLUTION

The skin is our number one defense against all environmental exposures. Air pollutants can lead to oxidative stress, which damages skin cells and accelerates aging.

DIET

Poor nutrition can affect the health and appearance of our skin. A diet lacking in macros (carbs, proteins, fats, fiber, and water) and micronutrients (vitamins and minerals) can lead to dull skin and exacerbate the signs of aging.

ALCOHOL CONSUMPTION

Excessive alcohol intake can dehydrate the skin and cause inflammation, leading to premature aging.

STRESS

Chronic stress can lead to hormonal changes and the production of free radicals, which can accelerate skin aging. We will also discuss this topic in Chapter 6: Help Your Self Stress Less (page 168).

SLEEP DEPRIVATION

Lack of sleep can affect skin repair processes, leading to dull, tired-looking skin and increased signs of aging. We will discuss this further in Chapter 5: Help Your Self Sleep So Good (page 146).

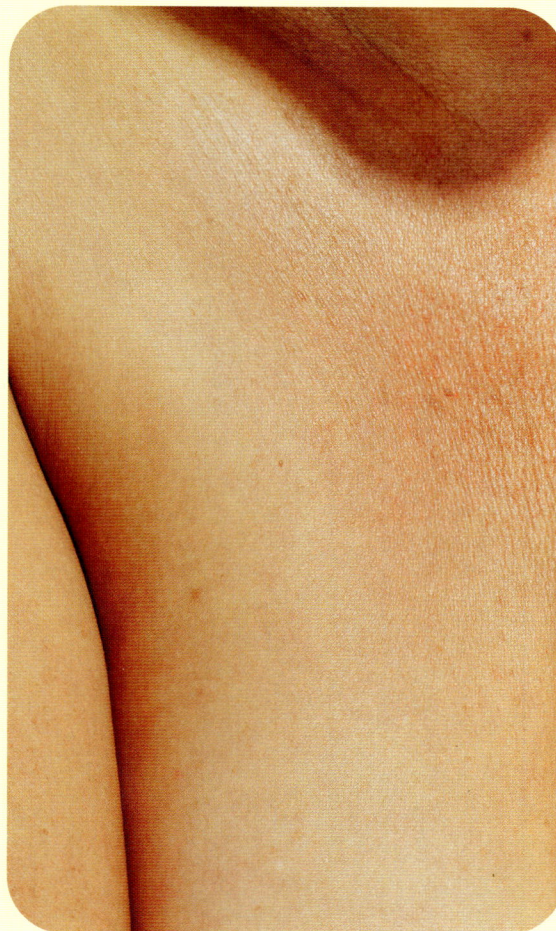

91

While intrinsic aging is inevitable, extrinsic aging is something that we can control through lifestyle choices, which we'll discuss throughout this chapter and throughout the book. Sun protection, hydration, healthy diet, limiting alcohol, having a regular skin care routine, sleep, and stress management—all these things benefit your skin, and we'll be covering them here.

Inflammation

Inflammation is an immune response that causes redness or swelling of an area of the body, and it's the body's natural response to injury or infection.

There are many lifestyle and environmental factors that contribute to inflammation, including chronic stress, poor diet and gut health, and disrupted sleep. Managing inflammation is critical as unmanaged inflammation increases the genetic expression of skin damage.

Your Skin and the Sun

Why the Sun Ages Us

The sunshine is our friend, boosting our vitamin D levels and keeping seasonal affective disorder at bay. However, soaking up too much of the sun's rays is incredibly bad for our skin. Sun damage to the skin occurs primarily through UV radiation, which damages DNA and breaks down collagen and elastin fibers. Excessive sun exposure (that's right, tanning!) accelerates the intrinsic aging factors and generates free radicals, leading to premature aging, wrinkles, and an increased risk of skin cancer.

And while there are plenty of reasons to exercise caution when it comes to sun exposure, we should not fear the sun. It's essential for good health. It regulates our circadian rhythm, and it's a great source of vitamin D, which is essential for bone, brain, and muscle health; immune health; and regulating mood and energy levels. We recommend daily, moderate sun exposure, and that you avoid sunburns at all costs.

The Great Sunscreen Debate

"I live in Southern California, and I wear sunscreen daily to reduce signs of photoaging, primarily on my face. But if I'm going to be out in the sun for an extended period, I rely on protective clothing, hats, and tents to protect my skin. Everyone's tolerance to sun exposure is different, but even if you're wearing sunscreen and not getting burned, you're still possibly getting too much UV exposure. Let the sun be your guide, not your enemy."

—MEREDITH

Undoubtedly, sunscreens protect against sunburn, reduce the signs of photoaging, and reduce the incidence of nonmelanoma skin cancer. However, despite greater use of sunscreens with UV filters over the last decades, the incidence of malignant melanoma is rapidly increasing. It may surprise you to learn that the evidence that sunscreens protect against malignant melanoma is mixed. This does not mean that you shouldn't wear sunscreen, but rather that it should not be your only line of defense.

Sunscreens are broadly divided into two categories: chemical sunscreens and mineral (physical) sunscreens. There's been a lot of discussion in the health world over which type is safer, with concerns raised about the ingredients in chemical sunscreens being endocrine disruptors and environmental pollutants. It's important to know the facts and take an informed approach when it comes to using sunscreen. **Let's break it down.**

The Best Way to Sunscreen

Sunscreen protects our skin by creating a barrier that absorbs or reflects UV radiation before it can damage the skin. The two primary (and most well understood) types of UV rays are UVB and UVA. UVB rays directly damage the cellular DNA, while UVA indirectly damages the DNA by producing reactive oxygen species (ROS).[5] There have been many recent advancements in sunscreen technologies, with options that are increasingly safe and effective.

When considering sunscreen, it's important to choose an option that:

- Is broad-spectrum sunscreen (offers protection against both UVA and UVB rays).

- Has an SPF (sun protection factor) of at least 30.

- Contains ingredients that are safe for humans.

- Contains ingredients that are safe for the environment.

Chemical Sunscreens

The Unsafe Six

Chemical sunscreens use active chemical ingredients to absorb UV rays and convert them into non-damaging heat. Chemical sunscreens are generally the most widely available, and they tend to be popular because they are lighter, clearer, and easier to apply than mineral sunscreens.

    The big concern with chemical sunscreens is over their ingredients, which may be unsafe for humans and for the environment. There has been a sunscreen cleanup in recent years, and there are now "clean" or "reef-safe" chemical sunscreens, meaning they are formulated with ingredients that are not known to harm humans or damage marine life. Both types tend to be mineral-based and promote transparency in ingredient sourcing and safety. With chemical sunscreens, we encourage you to be wary and avoid brands that include any of the chemicals deemed unsafe below. We always prefer a barrier sunscreen over a chemical (even "safe"); we'll discuss the distinctions below.

These are the six chemical sunscreen ingredients that you want to avoid at all costs. Be sure to read labels when considering sunscreen.

1. OXYBENZONE (BENZOPHENONE-3)

This is one of the most criticized sunscreen ingredients and has been shown to have endocrine-disrupting properties, mimicking estrogen with potential repercussions for reproductive and developmental health. It's also harmful to marine life. If you remember one ingredient to look out for and avoid when shopping for sunscreen, this is the one.

2. OCTINOXATE (ETHYLHEXYL METHOXYCINNAMATE)

This potential endocrine disruptor can cause skin allergies and contribute to coral reef bleaching.

3. HOMOSALATE

A potential endocrine disruptor that accumulates in the body, causing concern for long-term exposure. Also known to be toxic to aquatic life.

4. OCTOCRYLENE

This chemical ingredient breaks down into benzophenone, a known carcinogen. It's also harmful to aquatic life and coral reefs.

5. PABA (PARA-AMINOBENZOIC ACID)

Studies show the potential for DNA damage under UV exposure. PABA is not as widely studied, but it may cause harm to aquatic life.

The Passable Four

The following chemical ingredients are generally considered "clean" and safe. With that said, the idea of a "clean" chemical seems like a bit of an oxymoron to us, and there is plenty that is not fully understood.

    We prefer to use "clean" chemical sunscreens only occasionally in cosmetic applications where you might not necessarily be spending hours in the sun but need some aesthetically appealing coverage, such as tinted moisturizer or other cosmetic products containing SPF.

1. AVOBENZONE (BUTYL METHOXYDIBENZOYLMETHANE)

Provides broad-spectrum UVA protection. Generally nontoxic and non-irritating for most people.[6]

2. MEXORYL SX (ECAMSULE)

Exceptional UVA protection. Good safety rating and minimal risk of irritation.[7]

3. TINOSORB S (BEMOTRIZINOL)

UVA and UVB protection. Highly photostable and helps to stabilize other sunscreen ingredients. Generally considered to be safe.[8]

4. OCTISALATE (ETHYLHEXYL SALICYLATE)

Provides UVB protection. Helps stabilize other sunscreen ingredients. Low risk of skin irritation and toxicity.[9]

Mineral Sunscreens

Also known as physical sunscreens, these use natural minerals like zinc oxide or titanium dioxide to create a barrier on the skin's surface that reflects and scatters UV rays. Mineral sunscreens are widely considered to be safe. Zinc oxide and titanium dioxide offer broad-spectrum protection, pose little risk of irritation for those with sensitive skin, and are highly stable with little to no chemical breakdown. The downside of mineral sunscreens is that they have a thicker consistency, take longer to rub in, and may need to be reapplied more often. They may also leave a visible white film on the skin (picture the lifeguard with zinc oxide slathered on his nose).

Mineral sunscreen acts like a physical barrier against the sun's rays and it's our preferred choice, next to wearing protective clothing. Below are the ingredients that are commonly found in mineral sunscreens and are safe to use:

ZINC OXIDE

Broad spectrum, providing comprehensive protection through a physical barrier. Low skin irritation risk, high photostability, and no chemical breakdown.

TITANIUM DIOXIDE

Broad spectrum, providing comprehensive protection through a physical barrier. Photostable and no chemical breakdown.

IRON OXIDES

Primarily provides UVA protection. It has good photostability and helps protect against blue light.

KAOLIN (CLAY)

Mild UV protection. Gentle on the skin, often used to improve the texture of formulations.

SILICA

Scatters rather than absorbs UV light. Used to improve the texture of sunscreens.

MAGNESIUM OXIDE

Provides broad spectrum UV protection. Nontoxic and can provide other skin health benefits.

MICA

Reflects and scatters UV light, provides some level of UV protection. Adds shimmering qualities to makeup and cosmetic applications.

Iron oxides, kaolin, silica, magnesium oxide, and mica have been explored for their potential benefits in UV protection and cosmetic applications. They are typically used in formulations to enhance the properties of sunscreens and provide additional benefits like improved textures, oil absorption, and aesthetic appeal.

95

Apply and Reapply

"My husband will tell you how bad I am at applying sunscreen. He's often come to me with hand outlines on his back from poor application. I know I am not the only one guilty of this faux pas."
—MEREDITH

We can't emphasize enough the importance of proper application and reapplication of sunscreen. If you are going to be out in the sun for an extended period, a single application at 10 a.m. and then never again during the day won't cut it. This is an excellent way to burn if you are prone to burning. The science and efficacy behind most sunscreens depend heavily on how you use them, how much you apply them, and how frequently you apply them. This is not a case of setting it and forgetting it.

The safest form of sun protection: a physical barrier

"We think there is no shame in covering up to minimize sun exposure—looking a little wacky is worth it. A physical barrier of protection is the most clean and effective way to minimize excess sun exposure, and you can pull the layers back as needed."
—MEREDITH + KAT

By this point you've probably gathered that our favorite form of sun protection is one that involves zero potentially unsafe chemicals. When out in the sun, we're big fans of wide-brimmed hats, umbrellas, and protective clothing to provide a physical barrier against the sun. There are also an increasing number of clothing options with UPF (ultraviolet protection factor) coverage. We're not going to get into the weeds of sun protective clothing in this book, but we generally recommend natural, tightly woven fabrics. Darker colors also typically offer more sun protection than lighter colors.

How much sun is safe?

We are all different when it comes to the amount of sun that we can safely tolerate. How you react to sun exposure has many variables, including your skin type and texture, genetics and family history of skin cancers, geographical location, diet, and any medications you are on (as certain medications increase sun sensitivity). If you know that you burn rapidly within twenty minutes of being in the sun, then don't stay out in the sun for four hours, even if you are covered in SPF 100 sunscreen.

Science indicates that short and regular amounts of sun exposure are ideal for "safe" sunning, vitamin D synthesis, and immune-boosting benefits. The amount of sun exposure a person can tolerate varies depending on their skin type and geographical location: Experts generally recommend within the range of fifteen to thirty minutes two to three times a week for average skin types. Very fair-skinned people should only get about ten to fifteen minutes, and if you are darker skinned, thirty to forty-five minutes.

We recognize that for some this seems like a lot of sun, and for others it might feel like very little. Pay attention to your skin type, trust your gut, do what is right for your lifestyle, and avoid burning. Be especially mindful about sun exposure between 11 a.m. and 3 p.m., when the sun is highest in the sky and UV levels are greatest, meaning that unprotected skin can burn within minutes. Be sure to wear a hat and protective clothing when out in the sun during these hours.

Balancing the benefits of sun exposure requires a mindful approach and doing what feels right for you and your lifestyle.

Antioxidants for Sun Protection

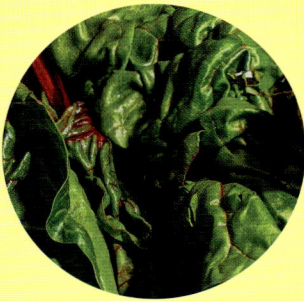

Studies show that a diet that is rich in antioxidants, in particular vitamins C and E, may provide better protection against the sun than sunscreen alone.

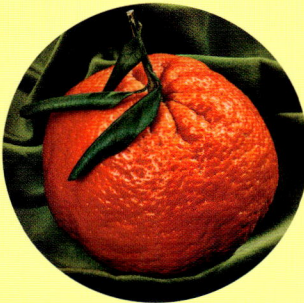

Foods rich in vitamins C and E, such as tomatoes, carrots, citrus, and dark leafy greens, are all wonderful sources of vitamin- and mineral-rich internal protection.

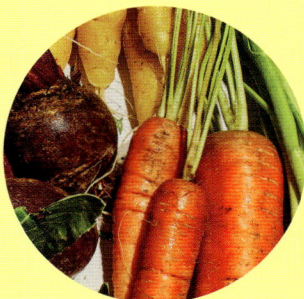

There are also high-quality supplemental forms of vitamins C and E available that have been shown to reduce sun sensitivity.[10]

SKIN CARE

Avoiding sun damage is probably the single biggest thing you can do for your skin to prevent premature aging. But what else is important? We're going to give you the facts on what is worth doing and what is worth skipping when it comes to topical skin care products, ingestibles, injectables, surface treatments, and more.

Hydrated, Moisturized Skin

Repeat after us: Hydrated, moisturized skin equals happy and healthy skin. This one may sound like a no-brainer, but the truth is that many of us seek invasive treatments, expensive topicals, and facials while neglecting the fundamental importance of properly hydrated, moisturized skin.

When the skin is hydrated and moisturized, its sensitivity is naturally reduced, and skin tone and texture improve. In fact, an advanced skin care regime will have little to no value if you don't start out with well-hydrated and moisturized skin. Not only will other topical treatments be less effective, but you could very well damage your skin if you use advanced technologies or aggressive exfoliants on dry and easily irritated skin.

The benefits of properly moisturized skin include:

• Improved skin barrier function, which helps protect against bacteria, pollutants, and other skin irritants

• Reduction in the visibility of fine lines and wrinkles

• Skin healing and repair support, reducing skin sensitivity and discomfort

• Enhanced efficacy of other skin care products

There are two main factors at play here: The first is **hydration**, which comes from drinking water, consuming it in water-rich foods, using a humidifier, and using externally hydrating products that act as humectants (products that draw water in) like hyaluronic acid, aloe vera, and glycerin.

The second factor is **moisturization**, which results from external application of skin care products that act as occlusives (preventing water loss). Think fats like oils and butters. Chapter 4: Help Your Self Hydrate (page 118) touches on skin, and many of the foods and lifestyle protocols work in tandem for skin health and proper hydration.

Tested Topicals

Topicals are skin care products applied directly to the skin to improve its appearance, and they come in many forms, including lotions, creams, gels, and serums. While many of the same ingredients are included in a wide range of product types, we generally recommend the serum form for the most concentrated and active ingredient applications. Serums have smaller molecules compared to moisturizers, allowing them to penetrate deeper. You don't always get what you pay for, but it is important to do your research when selecting serums containing potent topicals.

● Packaging: Look for airtight packaging in opaque containers that protect the ingredients from light, air, and moisture.

● Consider serums with ingredients that are known to work well together. For example, vitamin C and vitamin E are often combined for enhanced antioxidant protection, and niacinamide and hyaluronic acid together can improve skin hydration very effectively without irritation. Other ingredients stabilize each other, such as antioxidants (vitamin E or C) combined with ferulic acid, which can enhance the stability and efficacy of the serum. We advise you to focus on serums that contain minimal ingredients, and research their compatibility.

● Active Ingredients: Look for active ingredients. Many products with active ingredients will be labeled with percentages or concentration (e.g., "vitamin C 10%"). Be sure to check marketing materials and consult brand literature or a trusted source.

● Always be mindful of storage instructions and expiration dates.

Below is a list of topical skin care actives that are backed by science and have shown measurable results when applied to the skin. When using actives, we advise going slow and adding in one thing at a time to see how your skin reacts.

Retinoids (RETINOL AND RETINYL PALMITATE)

Retinoids are topical skin care products that have multiple benefits: they reduce fine lines and wrinkles, improve skin texture, stimulate collagen production, and treat acne. They work by increasing skin cell turnover, causing natural exfoliation. While retinoids can be very effective, it's best to first consult with a dermatologist before using retinoids, as they can irritate sensitive skin and should not be used during pregnancy and while breastfeeding.[11]

Vitamin C (ASCORBIC ACID)

Topical vitamin C has many benefits for your skin, including brightening skin tone, reducing hyperpigmentation, preventing sun damage, and stimulating collagen production. Topical products with vitamin C include everything from serums and moisturizers, to face wash and toner. We are fans of vitamin C serums as they typically have the highest concentration, deepest penetration, and offer the most stable format.[12]

Hyaluronic Acid (HA)

Hyaluronic acid is a substance that your body produces naturally. It helps your skin stretch, flex, and retain moisture. As we age, hyaluronic acid in our skin starts to disappear, contributing to the signs of aging. Topical hyaluronic acid is believed to work by hydrating and plumping the skin and reducing the appearance of fine lines. Hyaluronic acid can also be taken by mouth as a supplement and as a filler or injectable.

Niacinamide (VITAMIN B3)

Research also shows that niacinamide, or vitamin B3, has many skin benefits, including reducing inflammation, minimizing pores, improving skin elasticity, strengthening the skin barrier, and reducing hyperpigmentation. It is included in topical skin care products ranging from serums to cleansers. We recommend the serum form.[13]

Peptides

Topical peptide treatments have been shown to stimulate collagen production, improve skin elasticity, and reduce the appearance of fine lines and wrinkles. Although the research is relatively recent, and most peptides are pending FDA approval, the research is favorable for the efficacy of peptides.[14]

The Science of Ingestible Skin Care

Now that you've mastered the skin care basics, it's time to go a level deeper. As we've discussed, diet and nutrition are key factors in making sure that our skin looks its best as we age. If we want to maintain healthy skin and prevent premature skin aging, adequate water, protein, and micronutrient intake is critical.

And while it is entirely possible to get these elements through dietary sources, there are also an increasing number of ingestible beauty supplements on the market that research shows may improve signs of skin aging.

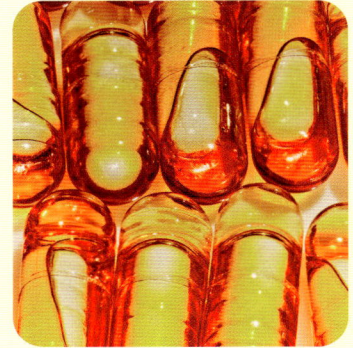

HYALURONIC ACID

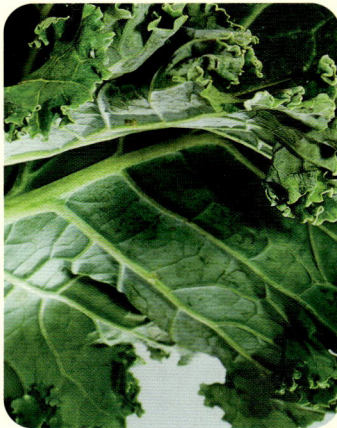

We discussed hyaluronic acid on page 99 as a key effective ingredient in topical skin care products. But did you know that research has also shown it to be beneficial as an ingestible product? Recent clinical trials reveal that ingestible hyaluronic acid, in pill form, supports skin hydration, smoothness, and radiance and may decrease the appearance of wrinkles. Low molecular weight is the most potent and scientifically sup-ported form of ingestible HA, known for its high bioavailability and effectiveness in improving skin and joint health.[15]

THE FOLLOWING FOODS SERVE AS GOOD DIETARY SOURCES OF HYALURONIC ACID:

- Citrus foods high in vitamin C
- Soy products
- Leafy greens
- Root vegetables

CERAMIDES

Ceramides are the main lipids in the outermost layer of the skin and are crucial for maintaining the skin's barrier. Our skin ceramides decline with age, and although studies are limited, positive results have been shown with ceramide supplementation. Human clinical trials show that ingestible ceramides derived from wheat may support skin hydration radiance and may decrease the appearance of wrinkles.[16]

THE FOLLOWING FOODS ARE ALSO GOOD DIETARY SOURCES OF CERAMIDES:

- Brown rice
- Soy products (tofu, edamame, soy milk)
- Wheat germ

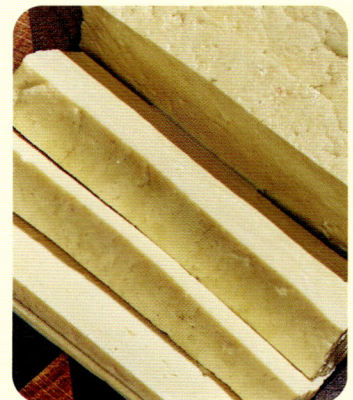

COLLAGEN

Collagen is the primary component of human skin. Collagen is an animal-derived protein, typically sourced from bovine, marine, or poultry origins, and some studies have shown that animal-based collagen supplements may work. The degree of effectiveness can vary widely based on the individual and type of supplement. While many people may assume that animal foods are inherently rich in collagen, this isn't strictly true. Collagen is derived from animal bones, skin, and connective tissue, not from the meat itself. Making bone broth is probably the most effective way to boost your collagen at home.

SIGNIFICANT FOOD SOURCES OF COLLAGEN INCLUDE:

● Bone broth

● Chicken and pork skin

● Skin, flesh, and bones of fish

● Cuts of meat with connective tissue

With that said, animal-based collagen isn't the only option.[17] If you are following a plant-based diet, you can boost your body's natural collagen production by consuming foods and supplements that support and boost the body's natural collagen production. Think of these products not as a collagen supplement, but as collagen-building support.

HERE ARE SOME COMMON VEGAN SOURCES AND INGREDIENTS USED IN COLLAGEN-BOOSTING SUPPLEMENTS:

● Vitamin C

● Amino acids (specifically proline and glycine). Building blocks for collagen, these amino acids can be derived from plant sources such as soy, quinoa, and legumes.

● Silica. Found in plants like horsetail and bamboo.

● Zinc. Pumpkin seeds and quinoa are both rich sources.

● Hyaluronic acid. In the synthesized supplementation form.

● Biotin. Found readily in nuts and seeds.

● Algae extracts. Spirulina and chlorella are rich in amino acids, antioxidants, and other nutrients that support collagen production.

FOODS THAT HELP THE BODY PRODUCE COLLAGEN INCLUDE:

● Citrus fruits

● Berries

● Leafy greens

● Beans

● Soy products

101

ANTIOXIDANTS

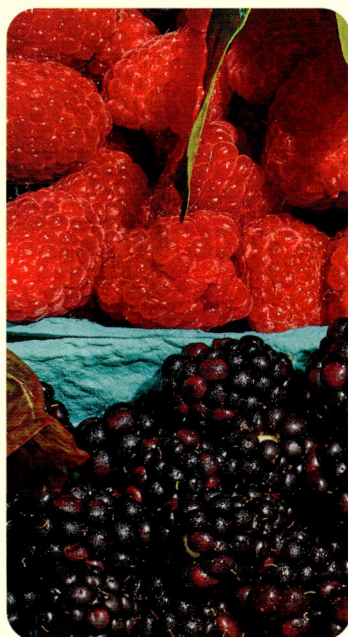

Antioxidants provide support against free radical damage. Dietary antioxidants may prevent DNA damage and tumor growth caused by UV radiation. Numerous studies have found that certain dietary antioxidants are promising in possible skin cancer prevention.[24]

THESE INCLUDE:

● Vitamin C

● Vitamin E

● Carotenoids

● Selenium

● Zinc

If you are eating a colorful diet that is seasonal and rich in diversity, chances are, you are getting a plentiful number of high-quality antioxidants.

HOWEVER, WE RECOGNIZE THAT THERE ARE CERTAIN FOODS WITH EXCEPTIONAL ANTIOXIDANT PROFILES:

● Berries

● Dark chocolate

● Spinach and kale

● Pomegranates

● Beets

● Beans

● Beverages like coffee and tea

YOUR

Your lymphatic system is located in the dermis, the second layer of your skin.

LYMPHATIC

It is a crucial part of the body's immune system and fluid balance.

SYSTEM

The lymphatic system helps regulate fluid in the body by collecting excess fluid (lymph) from tissues and returning it to the bloodstream. It plays a key role in the body's immune defense mechanisms by transporting white blood cells (lymphocytes) and filtering out pathogens, actions that are vital for immune function and detoxification.

What does this have to do with skin and aging? Proper lymphatic function can aid in maintaining the skin's structural proteins like collagen and elastin. Because of its location in the dermal layers, the flow of the lymph essentially helps combat some of the signs of intrinsic aging through nutrient delivery and support of the skin structure. So much of skin care has an external focus, but paying attention to lymphatic flow is a great way to tone your inner layers of skin. Studies have shown that lymphatic flow may help to keep the skin firm, elastic, and youthful looking. Effective lymphatic drainage can also help to unclog pores by removing the excess sebum and dead skin cells that can cause acne and other blemishes.

The primary role of the lymphatic system is to expel toxins from our body. **If our lymphatic system is blocked, this shows up on our skin in the form of acne, dryness, and puffiness.** Lymphatic drainage is the process of draining lymph from our lymph nodes by physically moving the lymph through the lymphatic system. The lymphatic system does not self-circulate like the cardiovascular system; therefore, you must do the work to drain the lymph properly.

There are straightforward, common-sense, and practical techniques out there for moving your lymph, all of which you can do on your own.

These methods include:
→ **Exercise**
→ **Dry brushing**
→ **Self-massage**
→ **Deep breathing**
→ **Hydration**
→ **Sauna/sweating**
→ **Avoiding tight clothing (tight bras especially!)**

We love to use our skin care routine as an opportunity to move the lymphatic system consciously through self-massage or dry brushing. When you apply body oils or lotions, we recommend focusing on and massaging the areas of the body that contain a dense amount of lymphatic tissue including the neck, armpits, and groin. To massage the lymph, it is generally recommended that you apply gentle pressure and use light rhythmic strokes toward the heart, starting with the neck and collarbone area and moving down to the arms, chest, and abdomen and then toward the groin area. You don't need to overthink these actions; being mindful of what feels good and natural goes a long way. This is also an excellent opportunity to check in on bumps and irregularities, and to understand what is normal for you and your breast tissue.

Our Favorite At-Home Skin Care Tools & Techniques

Dry brush for the body

If you've paid any attention to wellness culture over the past ten years, chances are you've heard of dry brushing. Dry brushing involves gently brushing the skin with a dry, natural-bristle brush in upward, circular motions toward the heart to exfoliate the skin and stimulate lymphatic drainage.

Simply start at the feet and use long, gentle strokes on your limbs and circular motions at the joints, moving upward. Brush in a way that feels comfortable and organic for you. It is an extraordinarily effective and accessible form of skin care.

It has been shown to have the following benefits:

- Exfoliation
- Improved circulation
- Lymphatic drainage
- Reduction in cellulite appearance
- Emptying clogged pores

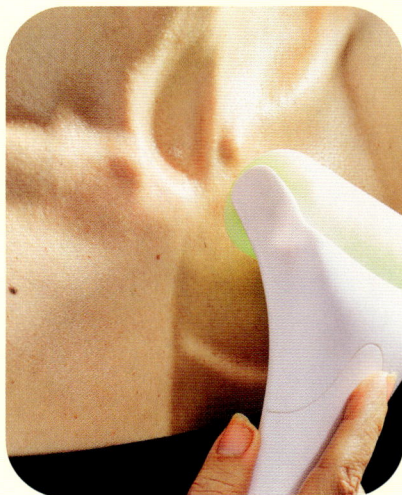

THESE ARE OUR FAVORITE TOOLS AND TECHNIQUES FOR AT-HOME SKIN CARE THAT ARE EASY TO DO AND PROVEN TO BE EFFECTIVE AND AFFORDABLE.

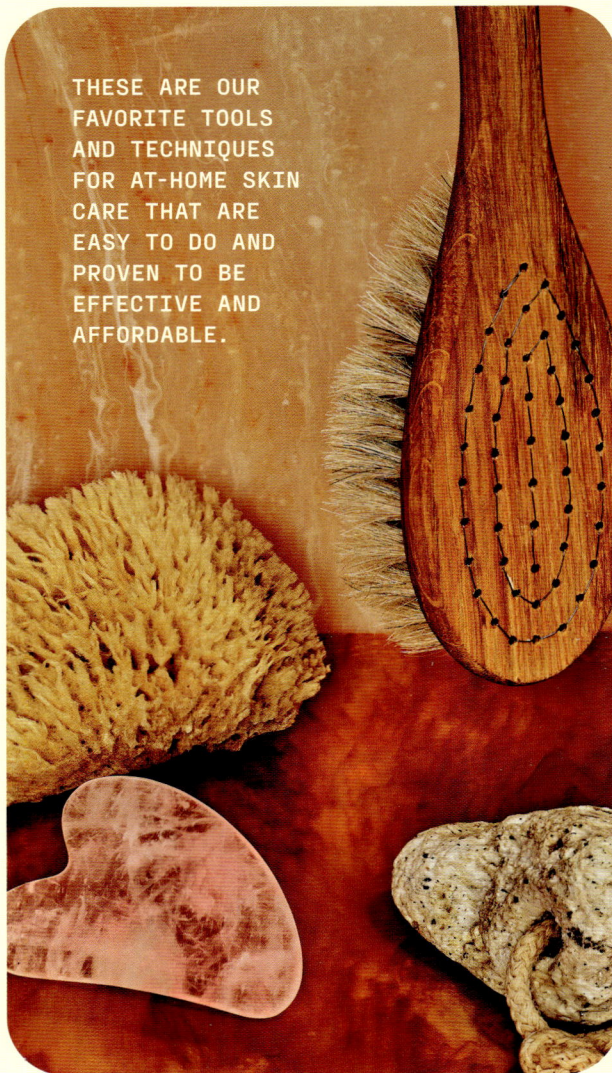

Ice rolling

"I'm obsessed with my ice roller. Sometimes I use it during the workday just to give myself a little pick-me-up."

—MEREDITH

Ice rolling is one of our favorite affordable and enjoyable skin treatments. It simply involves rolling a cold or frozen roller across the face to diminish puffiness, soothe inflammation, improve circulation, reduce facial tension, and sometimes help boost product absorption. Ice rollers can easily be found online for frequent use, or you can try freezing a cucumber to roll along your skin. We like to ice roll at night to help with the absorption of skin care products, but feel free to do it during the day too, if you're ever feeling hot and bothered.

Gua sha

Gua sha is a Traditional Chinese Medicine (TCM) technique that involves using a smooth-edged tool to apply pressure and scrape the skin. Gua sha works by increasing surface microperfusion, the flow of blood through the smallest vessels in the circulatory system, including capillaries, arterioles, and venules. Stimulating microperfusion through gua sha may improve blood flow and nutrient delivery resulting in improved skin, texture, and tone.[19]

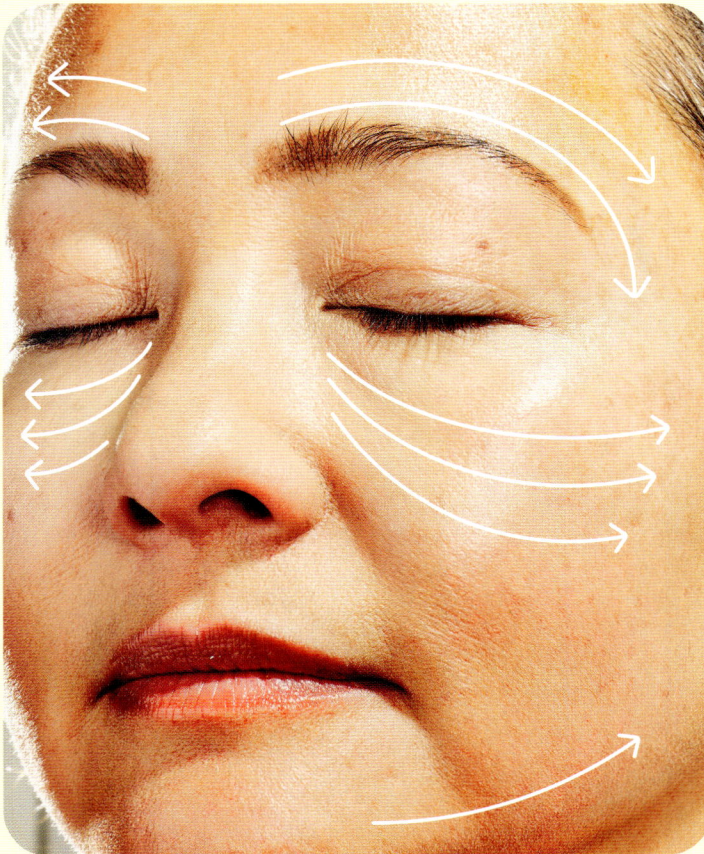

We recommend doing it on clean skin with a light oil or serum to help the tool move smoothly. Hold at a 15- to 45-degree angle, almost flat against your skin. Using light pressure, start at the base of your neck, moving upward toward your jawline. This helps promote lymphatic drainage and circulation.

Gua sha may provide the following benefits, and we've experienced many of them firsthand:

- Pain relief
- Reduced inflammation
- Immune support
- Relief of facial tension and puffiness
- Relief of sinus pressure

Facial massage

Often touted as the "natural facelift," facial massage kick-starts lymphatic drainage and improves blood circulation and skin elasticity. The technique involves using gentle, upward strokes starting at the jawline and moving up the face, to stimulate circulation, relax facial muscles, and promote a healthy, glowing complexion. Over time, it may lead to more defined facial features, reducing skin droopiness and the appearance of fine lines and wrinkles. The loss of blood flow in our dermal layers is one of the key factors in the skin aging process, and increasing blood flow with a technique like facial massage will have visible benefits.

Minimally Invasive Procedures for Skin Health

There are so many exciting new technologies when it comes to noninvasive skin care treatments. We believe that in ten years' time injectables will no longer be the norm—and enhancing skin longevity through treatments that fortify and amplify our skin's natural resilience will be the future.

MICROCURRENT THERAPY

Microcurrent therapy uses low- to medium-frequency pulsed electric currents to create an electric field that penetrates the skin. These electrical pulses stimulate deeper layers of skin, muscles, and tissue, resulting in antiaging benefits such as wrinkle reduction, skin tightening, and improved facial contours. It is believed that microcurrent stimulation, compatible with the body's natural electrical currents at the cellular level, enhances tissue repair, positively affects blood flow, and may help reduce epidermal thinning.[20]

LED THERAPY

The science behind LED therapies is solid, and many good at-home tools exist. LED therapy uses specific wavelengths of light to penetrate the skin and target cellular components, primarily mitochondria. This process enhances ATP production, modulates ROS, and activates genes involved in repair and regeneration, leading to various therapeutic effects such as antiaging, wound healing, inflammation reduction, acne treatment, and pain relief. The noninvasive nature and broad range of benefits make LED therapy a popular choice in both medical and aesthetic fields.[21]

RADIO FREQUENCY THERAPY

Radio frequency (RF) therapy uses high-frequency electric currents to heat skin tissue to enhance the skin's natural resistance. This targeted temperature increase alters the skin's collagen structure, stimulating new collagen and elastic fiber production. While lasers (and heat treatments) can often exacerbate melasma (skin discoloration) due to their high-intensity light waves, radio frequency tools use sound waves, which are less likely to trigger pigment changes. The heat generated by RF can effectively treat sagging skin without aggravating melasma.[22]

MICRONEEDLING

Microneedling is a safe, noninvasive cosmetic procedure that uses fine needles to create micro-injuries in the skin. These micro-injuries stimulate the body's natural wound-healing processes, resulting in various skin benefits that include improved skin texture and tone, reduction in fine lines and wrinkles, reduced pore size, and improved skin firmness and elasticity. Microneedling also helps with product absorption, so it can be very effective when used in conjunction with other topical treatments. Science also shows that it may be beneficial in treating scars, acne, alopecia, stretch marks, and more.[23]

INJECTABLES

First, we'll start by saying that injectable skin care is widely variable in its form and function.

Fillers and Botox have been, and are, extraordinarily popular. While both treatments are generally considered safe when administered by a professional, these treatments fill in for volume (filler) or reduce wrinkles by acting on muscle movement (Botox). Think of these as a temporary fix for whatever aesthetic concern you might be trying to address. These formats are not about building your skin quality over time, and may have undesirable consequences if you become overly reliant.

We prefer improving the quality of our skin texture and tone through minimally invasive microneedling treatments in conjunction with ingredients that have bio-stimulating effects.

There is so much information out there when it comes to skin care, it can be truly overwhelming. As busy moms, our skin care philosophy is that less is more. We like to keep it simple.

MEREDITH'S SKIN CARE ROUTINE

● **7:00**AM
I wake up and splash cold water on my face every morning, then apply a dollop of balm and a spritz of mist (or rose water). Keeping my face hydrated is my goal.

● **7:30**AM
I'm a night bather, not a morning shower person, but I usually take a very quick body rinse in the morning to get going and then lather my body in oil. If I work out, I wait to rinse until after.

● **8:00**AM
I always apply vitamin C serum and sunscreen before I leave the house. I don't really wear makeup, but if I do anything it's applying a tinted moisturizer after the sunscreen has absorbed.

● **10:00**AM
I keep rose water–based mist with me and spritz myself with it throughout the day to keep my skin refreshed and hydrated, even in the winter.

● **11:00**AM
If it's hot outside, I like to put on a cold gel face mask at my desk to increase circulation, brighten my complexion, and generally wake up my face. I keep this in the refrigerator and do it when I'm in the mood.

● **1:00**PM
Hydrating lunches are good for your skin and help maintain energy throughout the day. Lunch for me is typically built on salad, with lots of healthy fats, beans, seeds, and olive oil.

● **3:00**PM
I get microneedling treatments every four months. They have been a game changer for my skin and are the only thing I do outside of home treatments.

● **5–6:00**PM
My nightly wind-down routine starts around this hour. If I can, I love to get mostly ready for the evening before we eat dinner: the rice is in the cooker, beans are on the stove, and Mom gets to take a bath. I dry brush before I get in the bath. I always use my body oil in the tub to shave and moisturize; oils with water are a great way to keep your skin extra soft. If I have extra time, I'll use my microcurrent tool (I have the NuFace) before bed.

● **7:30**PM
After dinner, I do my skin care routine. I use a 0.1 percent retinaldehyde in combination with whatever hydration-boosting serum I'm trying. I try to use the most natural but effective products I can find. I then top that with my balm and spritz with my mist for extra hydration.

● **7:45**PM
If I have time, I always try to do a lymphatic massage in combination with stretching before crawling into bed.

● **8:00**PM
I'm obsessed with getting my body really cool before bed, which helps you sleep. So the last thing I do in the evening is ice roll my face and (sometimes) body.

● **6:00**AM

I try to always dry brush before the shower, even if it's very quickly.

● **7:00**AM (OIL WASH AND LYMPHATIC MASSAGE)

Following my shower, I give myself an oil wash, gently cleansing using oils instead of soap, and a brief lymphatic massage. I like using an oil such as sea buckthorn that works with sensitive skin.

● **7:05**AM

I'll use a microcurrent tool (like NuFace) to model the skin.

● **7:10**AM (HYDRATE AND PROTECT)

Next, I'll apply a number of hydrating skin care products, from lightest to thickest:

→ Hyaluronic acid to plump

→ Vitamin C to brighten and protect

→ Moisturizer or balm

● **7:15**AM (APPLY SUNSCREEN)

The final step in my morning skin care routine is to apply a good mineral sunscreen, after the other products I use have had time to set.

● **12:00**PM

I'll spritz with rose water and reapply sunscreen.

● **1:00**PM (EAT YOUR WATER)

For lunch, I'll eat a hydrating meal, knowing that many vegetables are mostly water. This is usually a big salad with greens, grains, and maybe some tempeh, tofu, or avocado.

● **3:00**PM (FACIAL TIME)

Once a month, I love a good facial or face massage. It releases tension from the jaw and any stuck energy and rebuilds collagen production.

● **7:00**PM (RESURFACING AND REPAIR)

My nightly routine involves using ingredients to resurface the skin and build new cells at night. These include: retinoids, AHAs (alpha hydroxy acids), peptides, and niacinamide (vitamin B3).

● **8:00**PM (TAKE SUPPLEMENTS)

I take my supplements before bed, because it makes me feel like I'm nourishing my body while I sleep. I like stacking, and I never forget my skin care or brushing my teeth, so I do all that at the same time. I take a supplement that Ritual makes that has a lower-molecular-weight hyaluronic acid and ceramide, glycolipid. I also use hyaluronic and ceramides for my topicals. So I like the idea of inside out and outside in.

Skin Care Order of Operations

(AKA PEMDAS FOR YOUR FACE)

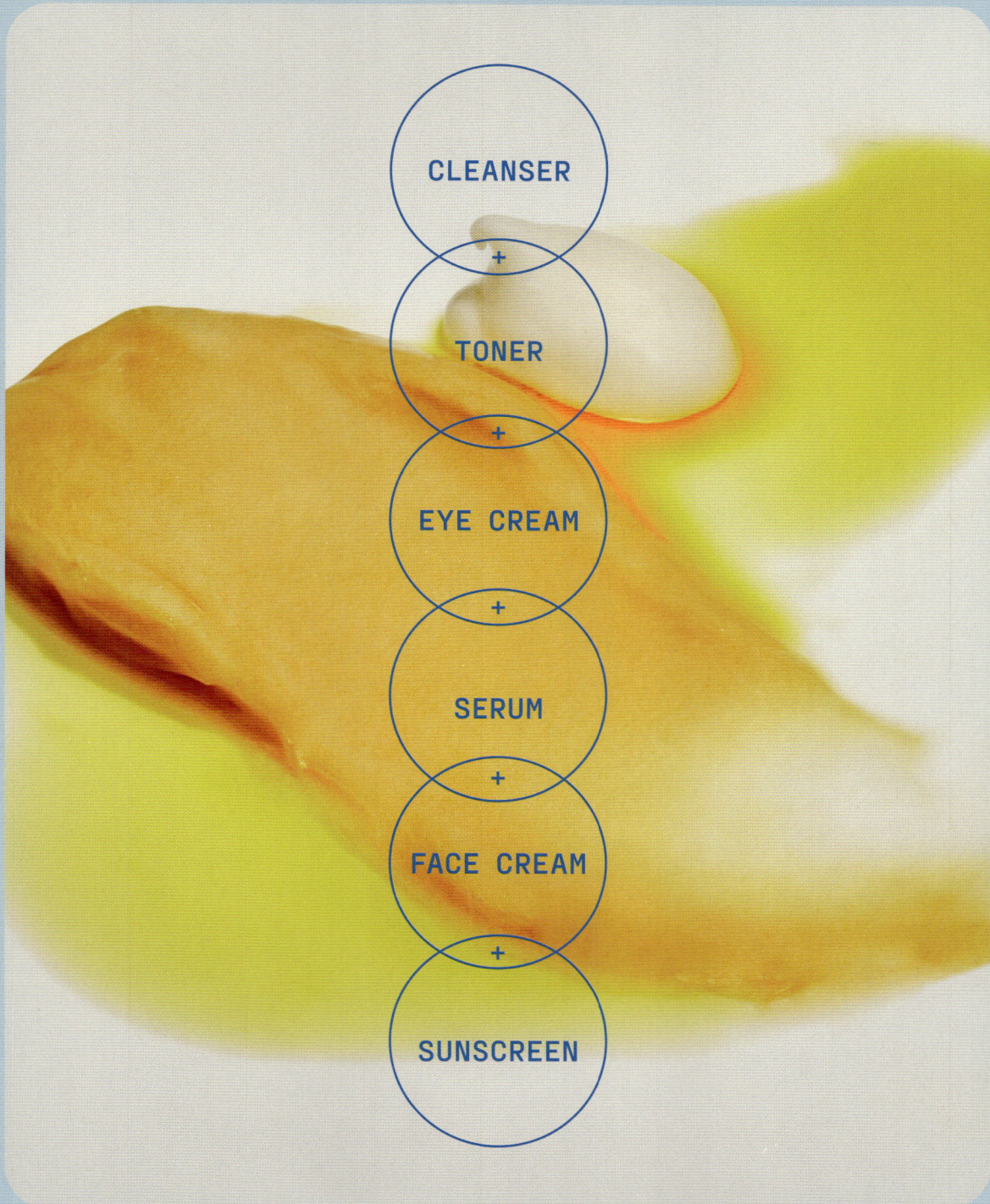

CLEANSER

+

TONER

+

EYE CREAM

+

SERUM

+

FACE CREAM

+

SUNSCREEN

The Recipes

Chapter 3

The ingredients in these recipes are a simple way to nourish your skin from the inside out. Packed with skin-loving nutrients, they support collagen production and boost natural hydration for a healthy glow. These foods are an easy and delicious way to give your skin the love it deserves.

→ **Brazil Nut, Dulse, and Golden Berry Snack**

→ **Sweet Potato Carpaccio**

→ **Lemon Coconut Bars**

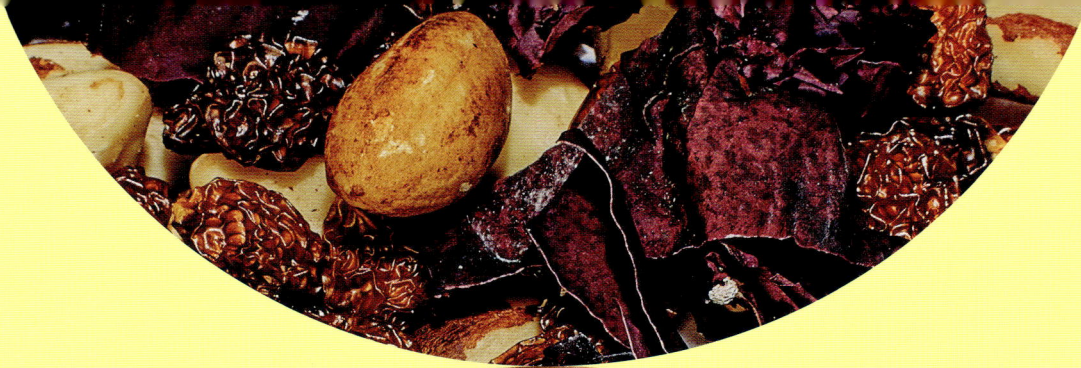

112

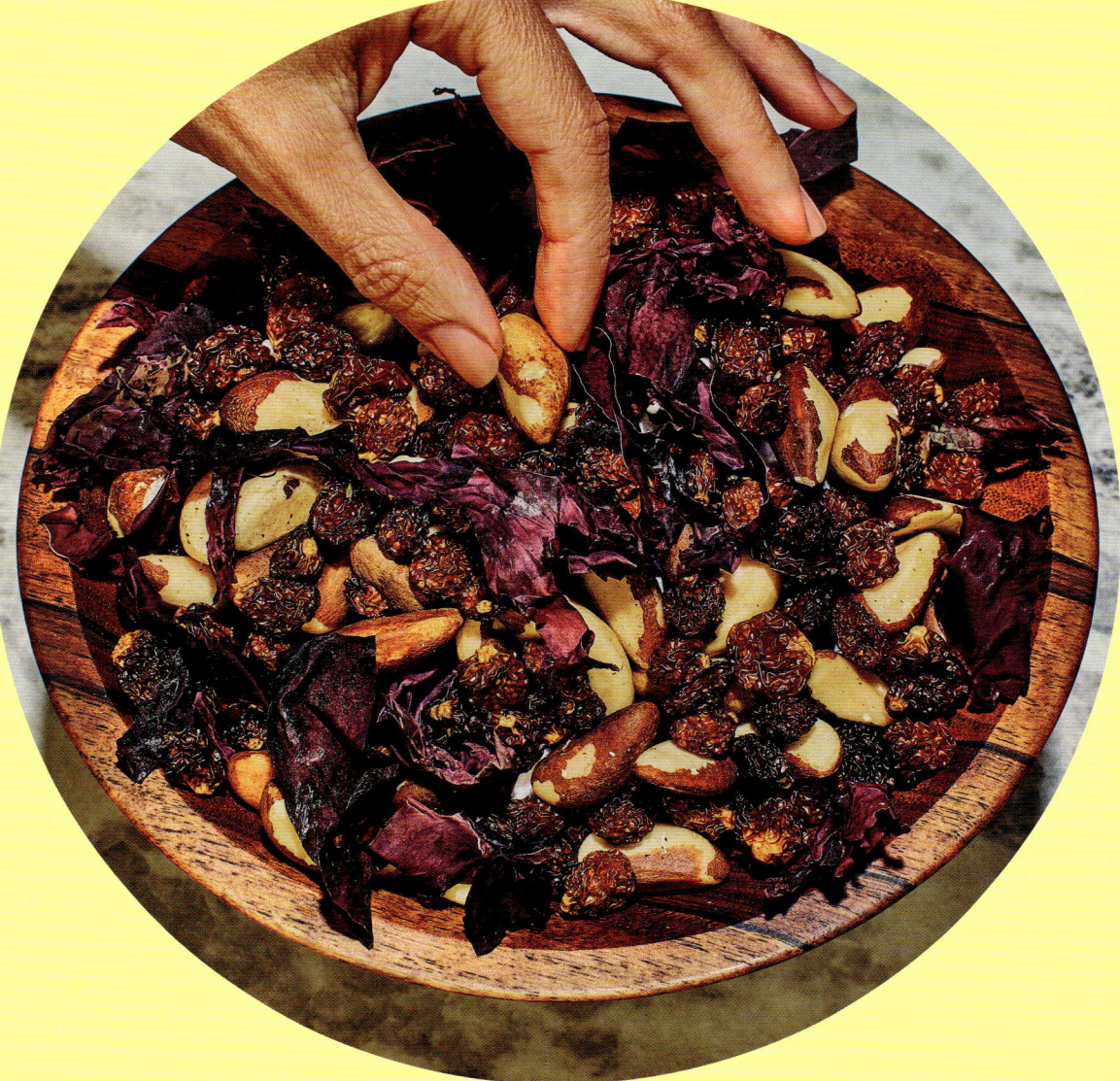

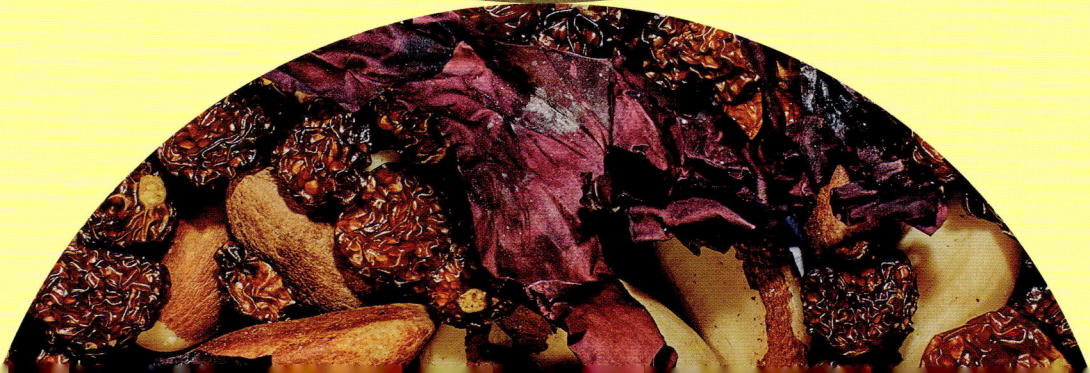

Brazil Nut, Dulse, and Golden Berry Snack

"One of my favorite anecdotes about the power of Brazil nuts features a gorgeous elderly woman I met in NYC who was eating a far-from-healthy diet but had radiant skin. Her beauty secrets were Brazil nuts and Vaseline. While I'd trade the Vaseline for my own balm, I took the Brazil nut recommendation to heart and started eating them regularly for their uniquely high selenium content."

—MEREDITH

MAKES ABOUT 2 CUPS (ABOUT 300 G)

1 cup (140 g) Brazil nuts

½ cup (30 g) whole dried dulse seaweed

1 cup (120 g) dried golden berries

1 tablespoon honey (optional)

Generous pinch sea salt

How to make?

Halve or quarter the Brazil nuts or leave them whole if you prefer. Using a knife or kitchen shears, cut the dried dulse seaweed into bite-size pieces.

In a bowl or airtight container, combine the nuts, seaweed, and golden berries and stir.

If you prefer a touch of sweetness, drizzle honey over the mixture and toss gently to coat.

Add an ample pinch of sea salt to enhance the flavors.

Adjust to taste.

Selenium is a powerful antioxidant that helps protect skin from oxidative stress and supports skin health by reducing inflammation and preventing damage from UV rays—thus this recipe is perfect for a chapter on aging well. This is a mineral-dense snack with a unique umami flavor that you can feel really good about eating! Dulse is high in iodine, golden berries are an excellent source of vitamin C, and Brazil nuts are one of the richest sources of selenium found in nature. This dish is great as a snack on its own or chopped up and served on oatmeal.

In this case we prefer eating our nuts raw. While roasting and salting nuts absolutely brings out flavor, it can alter the nutrition profile and does cause some nutrient loss. If you want to roast the Brazil nuts, go right ahead—but we prefer not to.

Sweet Potato Carpaccio with Hijiki Caviar and Tofu Crème Fraîche

Inspired by the sophisticated and classic combination of caviar, crème fraîche, and potato chips, this was one of the more elevated creations that I made right out of culinary school. At the time, most of the plating and concepts for vegan food were fairly casual, so this combination of flavors felt uniquely refined. I still make this dish, served with a glass of champagne, when I want to impress.

The nutritive plus side is that this dish is rich in beta-carotene, vitamin A, iodine, and other trace minerals. Virtually every component of the dish is a skin superfood. Sweet potato is rich in beta-carotene—the precursor to vitamin A. Hijiki is a small brown seaweed that is used commonly in Japanese cuisine, known for its exceptionally high iodine content, so it is great to eat in smaller quantities, as we've presented here.

114

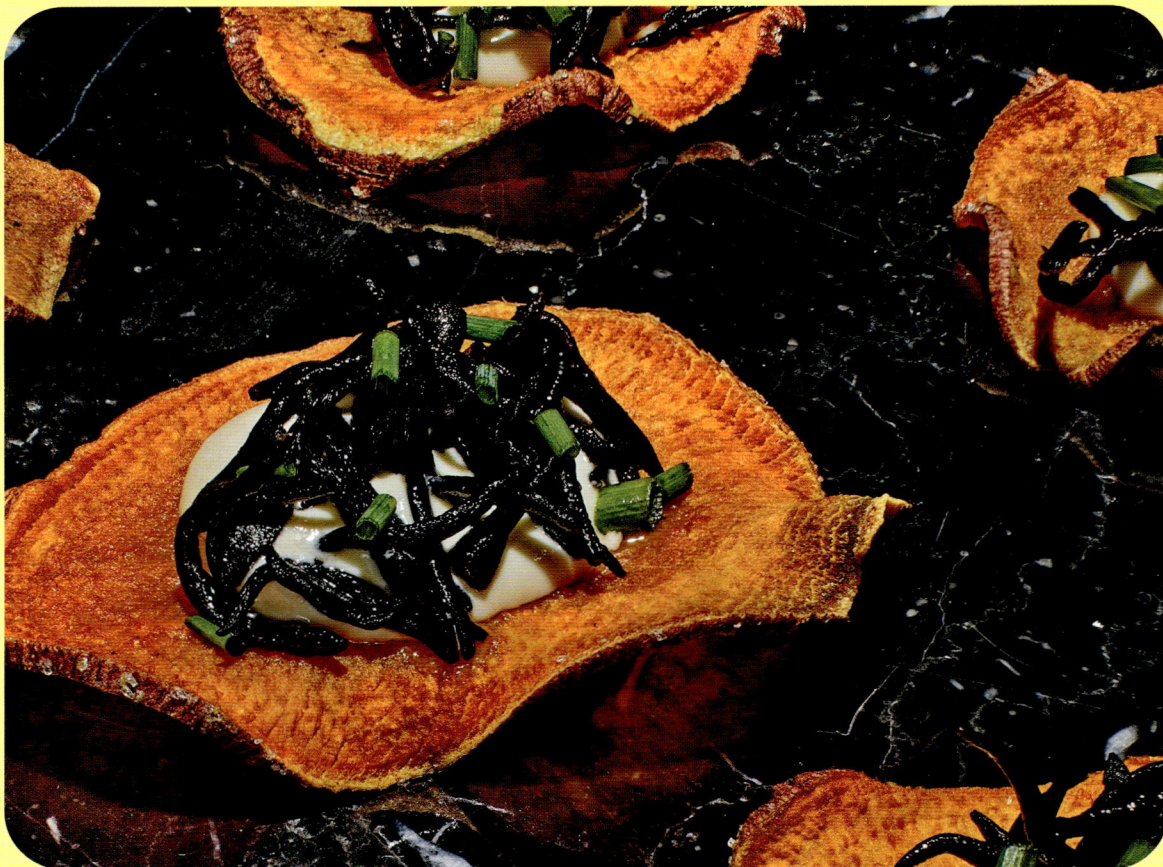

SERVES 6
AS AN APPETIZER

FOR THE SWEET POTATO CARPACCIO:

2 medium sweet potatoes

2 tablespoons olive oil, plus more for serving

2 teaspoons sea salt

FOR THE HIJIKI CAVIAR:

¼ cup (20 g) hijiki seaweed

1 tablespoon tamari or nama shoyu

FOR THE TOFU CRÈME FRAICHE:

1 (12-ounce/230 g) block silken tofu

1 tablespoon white miso

1 tablespoon fresh lemon juice

2 tablespoons olive oil

Salt and freshly ground black pepper

FOR GARNISH:

Chopped chives or microgreens

How to make?

→ Prepare the sweet potato carpaccio

Preheat the oven to 400°F (205°C).

No need to peel the sweet potatoes, but do so if you prefer. Use a mandoline or a sharp chef's knife to thinly slice them.

Put the sweet potato slices in a bowl, drizzle with the olive oil, season with the sea salt, and toss to coat.

Line a baking sheet with parchment paper, arrange the sweet potatoes on the parchment in a single layer, and bake for 15 to 20 minutes, until the edges are golden brown. Let cool while you prepare the crème fraîche and hijiki caviar.

→ Make the hijiki caviar

Fully submerge the hijiki in a bowl of water and soak for about 15 minutes until soft.

Drain, pat dry, and if desired finely chop the hijiki to resemble caviar. (If you love hijiki like we do, you can leave it whole.)

Toss the hijiki with tamari for elevated flavor.

→ Make the tofu crème fraîche

While the hijiki is soaking, in a blender, combine the tofu, miso, lemon juice, olive oil, and a pinch of sea salt and blend until smooth and creamy.

Add more salt and pepper to taste. Makes about 1 cup (240 ml). There will most likely be leftover crème fraîche, which can be stored in an airtight container in the refrigerator for up to 5 days.

→ Assemble

Transfer the sweet potato carpaccio to a platter, spoon the tofu crème fraîche over the top, and sprinkle with the chopped hijiki.

Drizzle with olive oil and garnish with chopped chives or microgreens.

Optionally, you can plate each sweet potato slice with an individual dollop of crème fraîche topped with hijiki caviar, to create individual bites.

Lemon Coconut Bars

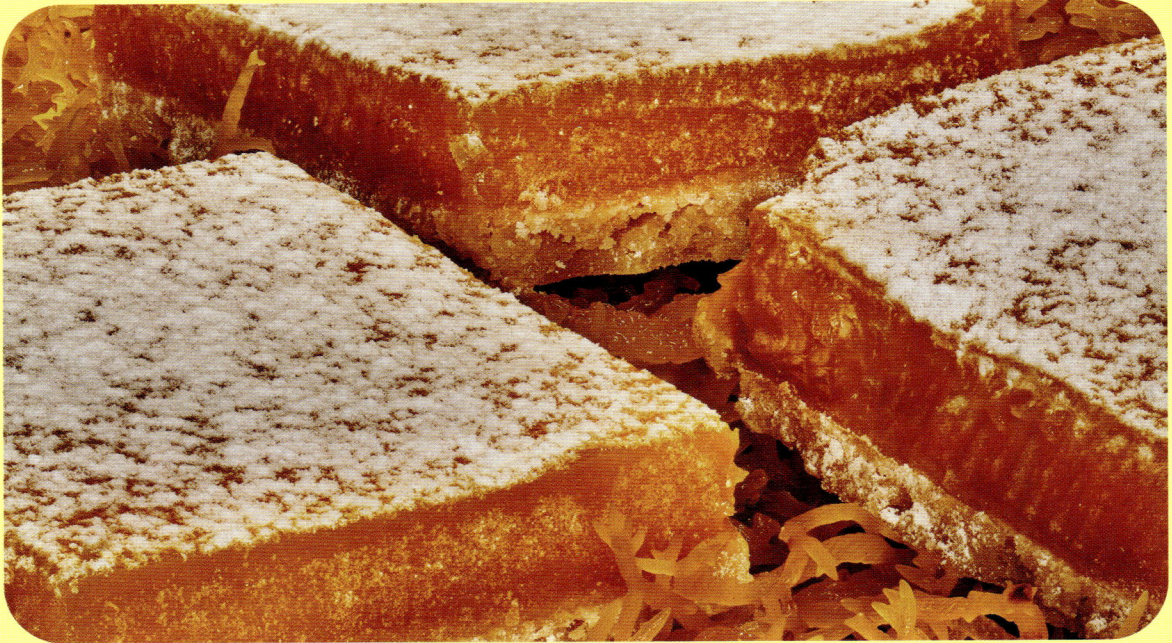

Although this recipe might be an entirely unfamiliar process, we promise the flavor won't be. The construction is a simple and sweet raw nut crust, made with a creamy and lemony filling using Irish moss instead of eggs. It has the sweet, tart flavor we all love in a lemon bar.

Preparing Irish moss can take some getting used to, but once you figure out how to incorporate it into recipes, it really can be a fun replacement for many dishes that have a gelatinous texture that would typically require gelatin or egg.

WHAT IS IRISH MOSS?

In the kitchen or applied externally, Irish moss, aka sea moss, can be beneficial to skin health. It has a nutrient-dense profile that is packed with vitamins A, C, E, and K, as well as minerals like iodine, calcium, and potassium, which help hydrate and nourish the skin. The collagen-like compounds in Irish moss may support skin elasticity and firmness. Its natural moisturizing properties can be used externally to soothe dry, irritated skin, and its anti-inflammatory and antimicrobial qualities may help reduce acne and skin redness.

Given that, in combination with all the vitamin C from the lemon in this recipe, we should probably call these bars a skin superfood.

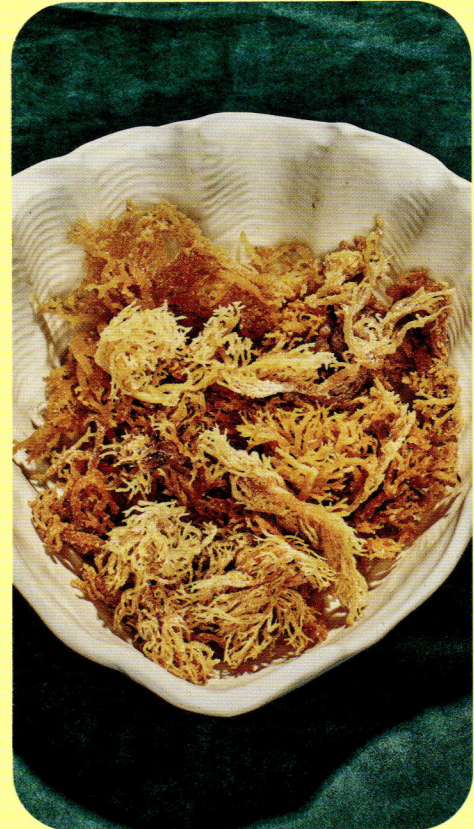

MAKES ABOUT 12 BARS
OR SLICES

FOR THE CRUST:

1½ cups (180 g) walnuts or
pecans

½ cup (45 g) unsweetened
shredded coconut

2 tablespoons coconut oil,
melted and cooled

2 tablespoons maple syrup

1 teaspoon pure vanilla
extract

Generous pinch sea salt

FOR THE LEMON
FILLING:

1 cup (120 g) raw cashews,
soaked in water for at least
4 hours or overnight

½ cup (30 g) Irish moss gel
or paste, store-bought or
homemade (made from
2 ounces/55 g Irish moss)

½ cup (120 ml) fresh lemon
juice

⅓ cup (75 ml) maple syrup

¼ cup (60 ml) coconut oil,
melted and cooled

1 teaspoon lemon zest

1 teaspoon pure vanilla
extract

Pinch sea salt

OPTIONAL GARNISHES:

Flaked unsweetened
coconut, pulsed in a food
processor to create a fine
powder

Zest of 1 lemon

How to make?

→ Make the crust

If you have a 9-inch (23 cm) square springform pan, now is the time to use it. If not, the 9½-inch (24 cm) round version will be fine. Line the bottom of the pan with parchment paper.

Pulse the nuts with the coconut flakes in a food processor to create crumbs. Do not over-blend; the mixture should not be sticky or smooth.

Add the melted coconut oil, maple syrup, vanilla, and sea salt and pulse until well combined.

Scatter the crust crumbs evenly over the bottom of the pan before pressing them down to ensure equal distribution. Chill in the refrigerator while preparing the filling.

→ Make the lemon filling

If you're making your own Irish moss gel, do so as described in the Tip.

Drain the cashews and pat dry.

In a high-speed blender, combine the cashews, Irish moss gel, lemon juice, maple syrup, melted coconut oil, lemon zest, vanilla, and sea salt. Blend on high speed until the mixture is smooth and creamy. Taste, and feel free to add a touch more vanilla, lemon, and maple syrup.

When blending, you want the texture to have a semi-thick pudding-like consistency. You need enough liquid to blend until the mixture is smooth but not runny. Depending on the Irish moss you are using, you may need to add a little more gel.

Pour the lemon filling over the crust and spread it in an even layer. Refrigerate for at least 4 hours or until the filling is set.

Remove the lemon bars from the refrigerator. Sprinkle with the powdered coconut and lemon zest, if using.

Remove the sides of the springform pan, slice the lemon bars into squares or wedges, and serve.

→ Tip: how to prepare Irish moss gel

When using Irish moss, it is important to rinse it thoroughly to remove sand and any other ocean residue. Once the moss is rinsed, cover with water and soak for at least 15 minutes, then rinse thoroughly.

Blend equal parts of the moss and water to create the Irish moss gel. Leftover gel can be stored in the refrigerator for up to one week to use in smoothies and other dessert preparations.

For this recipe we recommend blending about 2 ounces dried whole Irish moss (not flakes) with about ½ cup water. Add extra water to blend as needed.

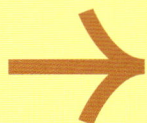
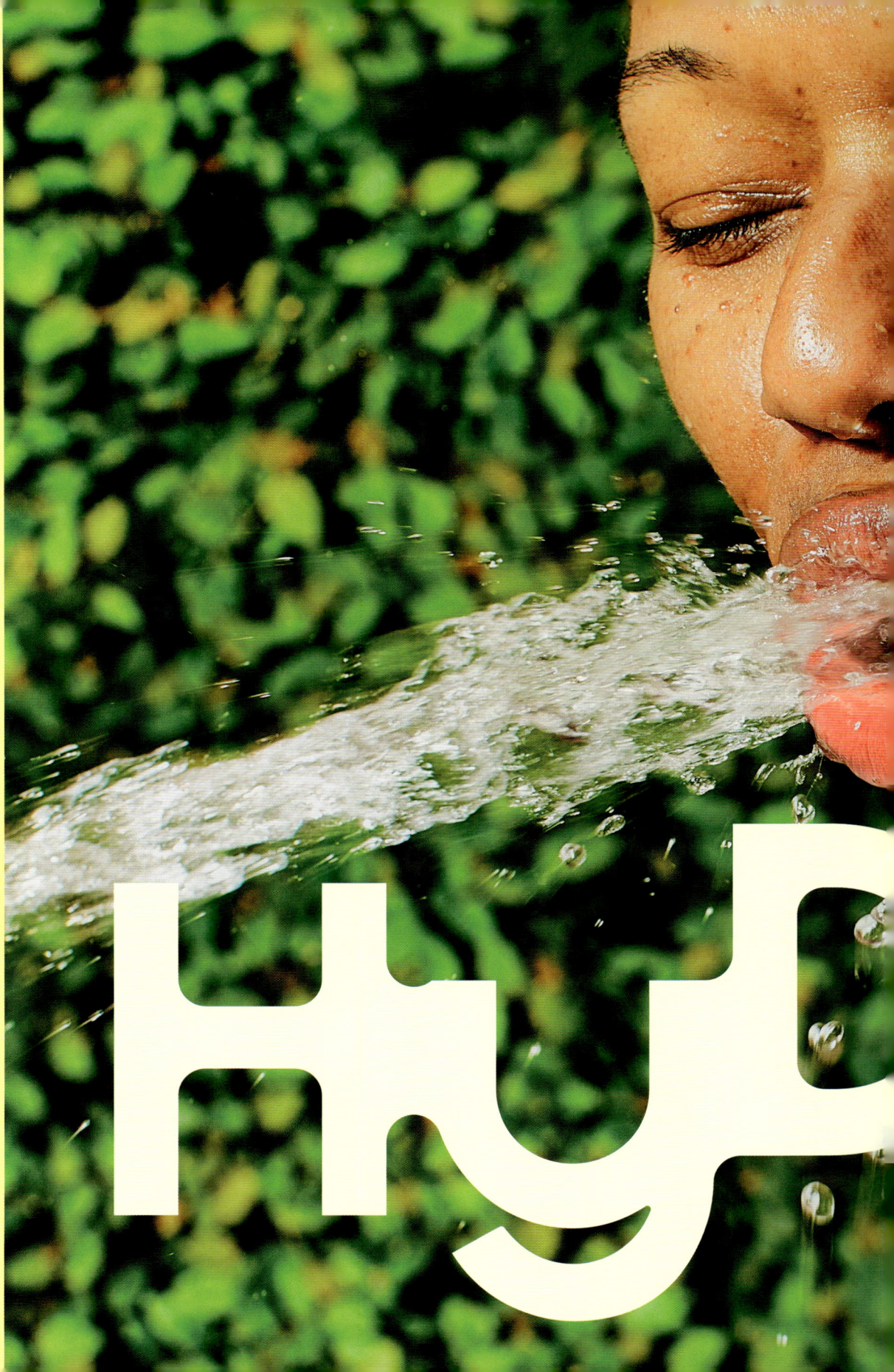

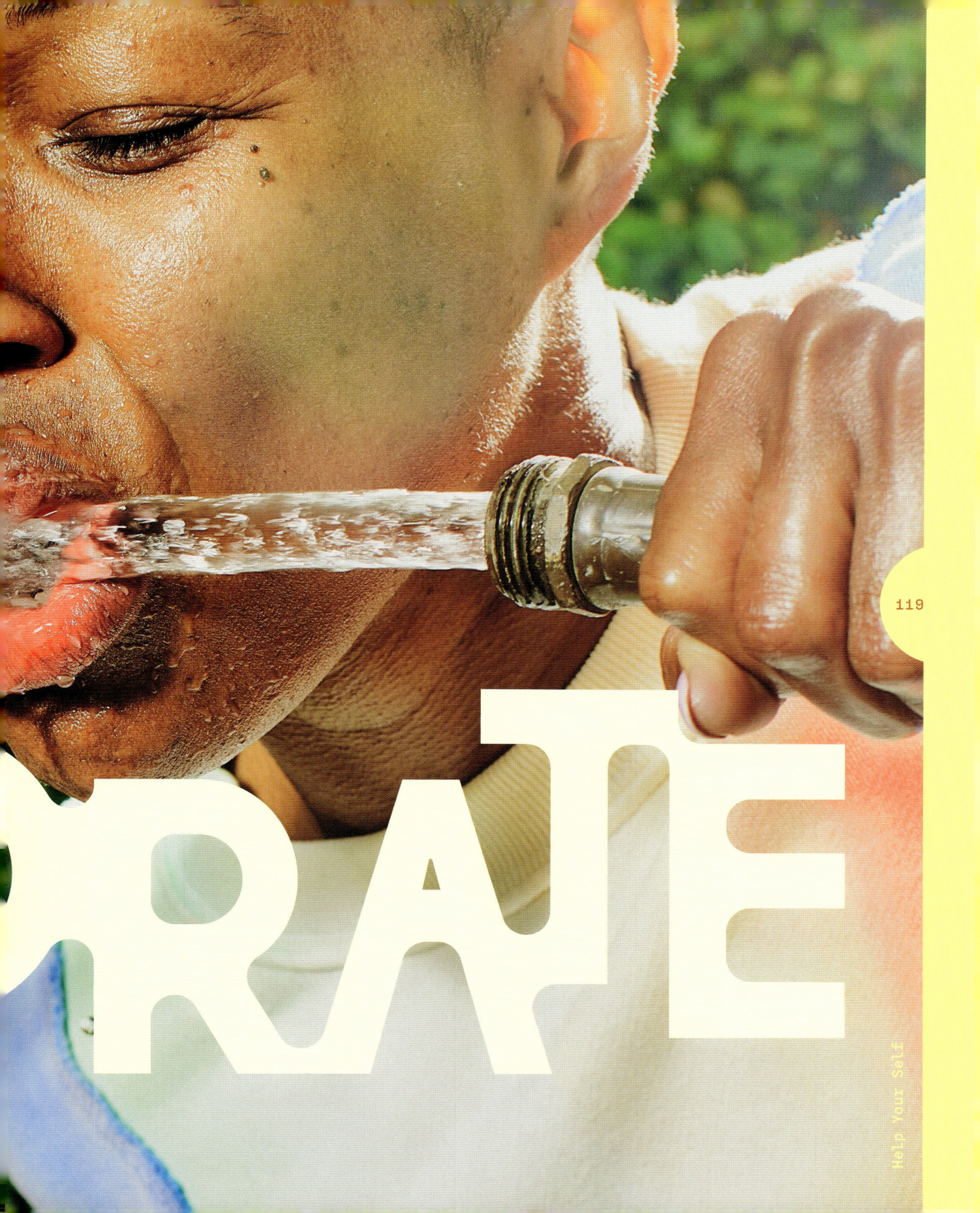

RATE

"My dad once showed up at my house with a water quality tester, and without telling me, he tested our water and determined that it wasn't safe enough to drink. He installed a new filtration system and changed the way I thought about heavy metals and contaminants in water. Once you start drinking properly filtered water, you realize that not only is it better for your health, but you can really taste the difference." —KAT

We are all obsessed with hydration these days, and the business of water has gotten a bit out of control. We walk around with water bottles that are comically large and are marketed like fashion accessories. Store shelves are lined with more flavored and bottled waters than anyone could ever need. But are we more hydrated? How much water do we really need? And what is the best type of water to drink? These are the questions we are asking ourselves, because not all of it is a gimmick. Hydration is one of the key factors of overall good health. When we are properly hydrated, things start to flow better. None of the advice in this book will truly be effective within a dehydrated body.

We recognize that having access to clean water is not a guarantee, even here in the US. If you are curious about your city's municipal water supply, you can check water quality by zip code on the Environmental Working Group's online database.

In this chapter, we're going to address the myths and lay out the facts when it comes to how much water we need to survive, thrive, and look and feel our best.

Why We Need Water

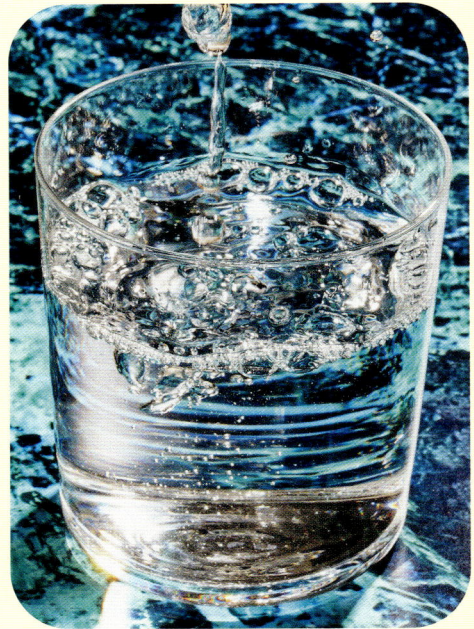

Water is essential to every one of our biological systems. The human body is made up of approximately 60 percent water, and water plays a vital role in all our bodily functions, including:

- Digestion and waste removal
- Temperature regulation
- Joint lubrication and maintaining skin elasticity
- The functioning of our senses
- Nutrient and oxygen transport

We are constantly losing fluids through sweating, exhaling, and waste elimination, and we need to constantly replenish these fluids in the body by drinking and eating—aka hydration. Staying hydrated is essential for health for so many reasons, some of which you may not have even considered.

• Hydration for brain health

Mental health is finally being addressed more, but hydration is rarely a part of that conversation. We believe that it should be. The brain is made up of about 75 percent water, and proper hydration is necessary for maintaining its structural integrity and biochemical processes.[1]

Regardless of what you are doing to address your mental health, you will want to make sure that your brain is hydrated, to improve:

CONCENTRATION AND MENTAL PERFORMANCE

Water helps transport oxygen and nutrients to brain cells, removes waste, and supports neurotransmitter function, all essential in supporting brain health and optimization. Dehydration can negatively impact cognitive functions such as attention, memory, and concentration.[2] The next time you can't focus and want to reach for another cup of coffee, have a glass of water instead.

MOOD

Hydration levels can influence mood and energy. Studies have shown that even mild dehydration can cause decreased cognitive performance and increased irritability due to elevated cortisol levels.[3]

• Hydration for detoxification and disease prevention

Proper hydration is essential to the body's natural detox pathways, supporting kidney, liver, digestive, and cellular function.

It's important to stay hydrated to improve:

KIDNEY FUNCTION

The kidneys use water to filter toxins and waste products from the blood, which are then excreted in urine, preventing kidney stones and urinary tract infections.[4]

CARDIOVASCULAR HEALTH

The heart requires water to function optimally and maintain blood volume and pressure.[5] Electrolytes are minerals in your blood and other bodily fluids that carry an electrical charge and regulate the heartbeat. When we are dehydrated, electrolyte imbalances can occur, leading to irregular heartbeat (arrhythmia) and other cardiovascular issues.

• Hydration for skin health

If we had to guess at why and how the water bottle became a status symbol, we'd bet that it has to do with skin health. While water isn't exactly the fountain of youth, staying hydrated has so many benefits for the skin.

We've already discussed this at length in Chapter 3: Help Yourself Age Well (page 86), but to recap, these are our top reasons to hydrate for skin health:

MOISTURE AND ELASTICITY

Hydration helps maintain skin moisture and elasticity, strengthening the skin barrier as an indispensable layer of protection. When the skin barrier is disrupted, it becomes more susceptible to environmental allergens, irritation, and symptoms of atopic dermatitis.[6] Not only does hydration improve appearance through moisture and elasticity, but it also serves an important role in the skin's overall health.

HEALING AND REPAIR

Proper hydration makes the skin more durable, allowing it to heal faster. Hydrated skin is also more responsive to antiaging treatments and products.[7]

• Hydration for performance

Hydration is crucial for physical performance to support:

EXERCISE

It's crucial to restore fluid balance before, during, and after exercise, replacing what was lost in sweat with fluids containing electrolytes.[8]

MUSCLE HEALTH

Proper hydration supports muscle function and prevents cramps by helping the muscles expand and contract properly. It also supports energy production, allowing muscles to perform at their best. Water also helps remove metabolic waste like lactic acid from muscles, reducing soreness and promoting faster recovery.

So how much water do we need?

We've all heard the advice about drinking eight 8-ounce glasses a day. And honestly, it's still a fine rule to follow, but it is by no means an absolute.

When determining your optimal water intake, it's important to consider personal lifestyle factors. If you are a long-distance runner, and you regularly use a sauna, you will need to be drinking substantially more water (and electrolytes) than your neighbor who isn't doing these things.

The official recommendations for water consumption vary a bit depending on who you ask, and they seem to have gone up a bit since the 8 × 8 (8 ounces of water 8 times a day) recommendation was first established.

Still, a general rule of thumb is between 1.5 and 3 liters (51 and 101 ounces) per day, depending on your personal needs.

This daily water allowance can come from beverages and from the foods you eat (more on that later in this chapter).

What Counts as Water?

Water isn't the only liquid that counts. To some extent, all liquids count toward your daily water intake, whether you are sipping on sparkling water (more on this on page 134), milk, sports drinks, or smoothies. Even coffee and tea count toward your liquid intake, though these two have mild diuretic effects, and we would never recommend drinking them in place of water for multiple reasons.

Plain filtered water is generally considered the most effective and straightforward option for hydration, because our cells can use it most efficiently and you aren't introducing additives, sugars, electrolytes, or other compounds that might be beneficial in certain situations but may delay absorption. Sparkling water is one exception, as the difference in absorption between sparkling and flat water is minimal. However, carbonation may cause issues for some people.

One big myth surrounding hydration is that coffee is extremely dehydrating. This is simply not true. Moderate consumption of coffee does not inherently cause dehydration. Alcohol is the one beverage that does dehydrate and that does not count toward your daily liquid intake.

Our take is that the best form of hydration comes from clean drinking water and eating water-rich foods. We'd recommend getting at least half of your daily liquid intake from plain water. It's just that simple.

123

"Eating hydrating foods hits differently. Just like you can't exercise your way out of a bad diet, I don't believe you can gulp water down to cover up bad eating habits. It just doesn't work that way. When I eat a water-rich diet—as cliché as it may sound—I see the difference in all aspects of my skin, digestion, energy levels, and mood. All the minerals and antioxidants that are swimming around in raw foods and juices . . . well . . . I believe they can do something good!"

—MEREDITH

When you eat a hydrating diet, everything changes. You'll find that you feel less thirsty (a given), that your digestion improves, that your skin may look better, and that you generally have more energy. By following a hydrating diet, you should be able to get about 20 percent of your daily water from water-rich produce and dishes like soups, stews, and salads. The amount of liquid you need to drink could also be substantially less than someone who is not eating water-rich foods.

124

EAT YOUR WATER

Here are some of our favorite water-rich foods:

- **CUCUMBERS**
  Approximately 95% water
- **LETTUCES**
  Approximately 95% water
- **TOMATOES**
  Approximately 94% water
- **ZUCCHINI**
  Approximately 94% water
- **WATERMELON**
  Approximately 92% water
- **STRAWBERRIES**
  Approximately 91% water
- **CANTALOUPE**
  Approximately 90% water
- **PEACHES**
  Approximately 89% water
- **ORANGES**
  Approximately 86% water

The beauty of this list is that the most water-rich fruits and vegetables naturally grow in the summer months (with the exception of oranges). It's as if nature knows we need these foods when it's warmer—because we do.

Our Favorite Produce in Season

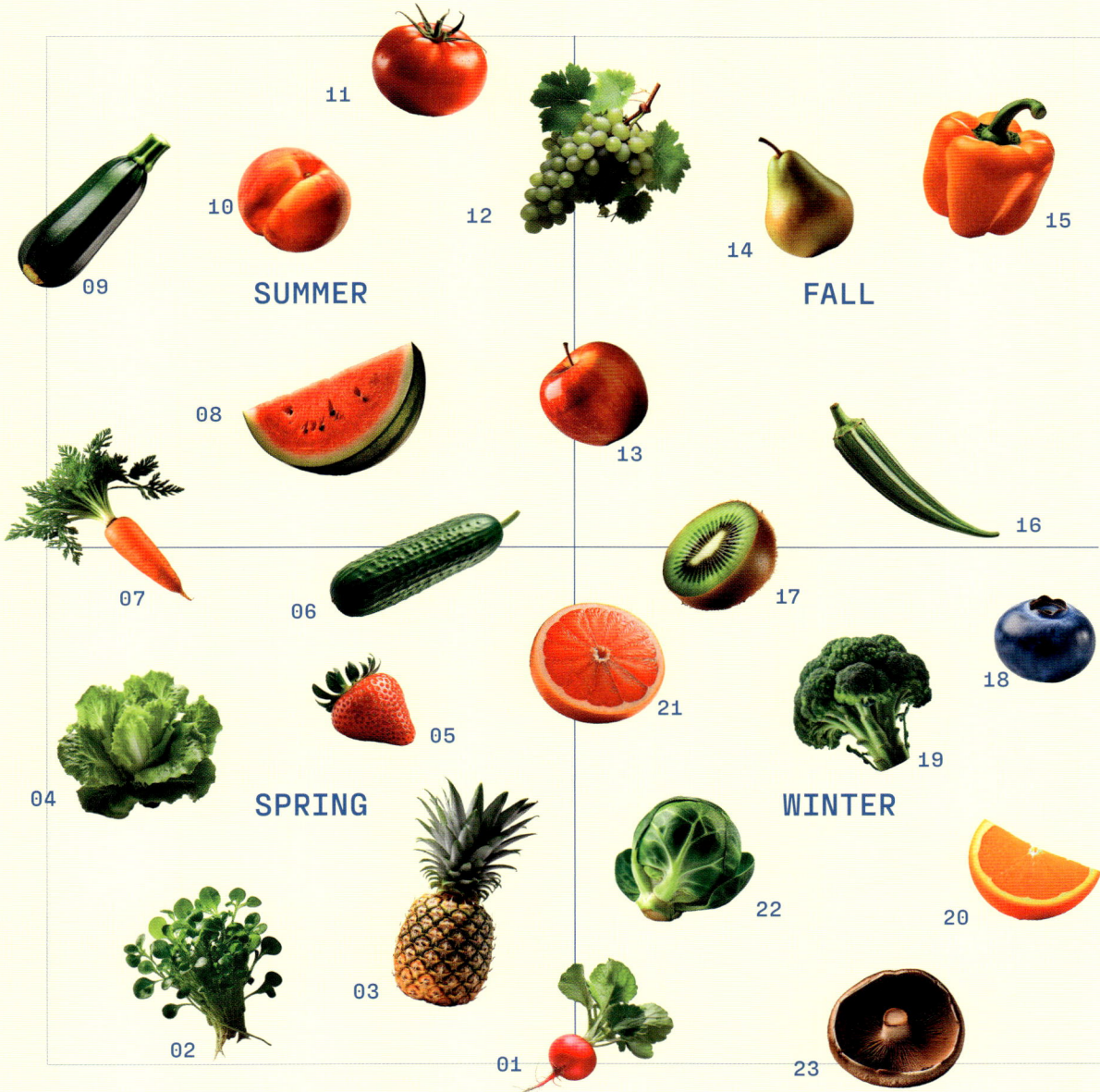

SUMMER

FALL

SPRING

WINTER

11

10

09

12

14

15

08

13

16

07

06

17

04

05

21

19

18

02

03

01

22

20

23

125

1. RADISHES	7. CARROT	13. APPLE	19. BROCCOLI
2. WATERCRESS	8. WATERMELON	14. PEAR	20. ORANGE
3. PINEAPPLE	9. ZUCCHINI	15. BELL PEPPER	21. GRAPEFRUIT
4. LETTUCE	10. PEACH	16. OKRA	22. BRUSSELS
5. STRAWBERRY	11. TOMATO	17. KIWI	SPROUTS
6. CUCUMBER	12. GRAPES	18. BLUEBERRIES	23. PORTOBELLOS

When do I need to up my water intake?

Thirst and urine color are good general indicators of proper hydration. If your pee is transparent to light yellow, you're probably hydrated, whereas if your pee is dark yellow, you may be dehydrated. But we can't always rely on this.

Other factors, such as your environment, play a role. If you live in a hot climate where you are losing a lot of water through sweat, you will need more daily water. Activities that cause perspiration, like strenuous exercise, also require more water intake.[9] The general recommendation is to consume 8 to 10 ounces of water for every fifteen minutes of strenuous exercise.[10] With light exercise, you probably don't need to replace as much additional water.

Women who are pregnant need an additional 10 ounces of water per day, and those who are breastfeeding need an extra 20+ ounces per day.[11]

Illness is another factor that can increase water needs. Fever, vomiting, and diarrhea can dehydrate us, significantly increasing our water needs by as much as 1 to 2 additional liters per day. The exact amount will depend on your individual needs,[12] so use your judgment and follow the direction of your health care provider when sick.

	HYDRATED
	IDEAL
	GOOD
	FAIR
	LIGHTLY DEHYDRATED
	DEHYDRATED
	VERY DEHYDRATED

What's with electrolytes?

Far beyond just drinking water, the science of hydration is all about electrolytes. In simplest terms, an electrolyte is a substance that breaks up into ions when dissolved in body fluids or water. These ions have electrical charges, and the differences in electrical charges in different body parts help move nutrients into cells, move waste, keep body fluids and blood pressure stable, and contribute to proper nerve, muscle, heart, and brain function. Essential electrolytes in our bodies include sodium, potassium, calcium, magnesium, chloride, bicarbonate, and phosphates.

Our bodies absorb electrolytes through food and drink and, in turn, expel them through sweat, urine, and waste. If we're not replacing those electrolytes—especially during strenuous exercise or hot weather—the equation can become imbalanced, leading to symptoms of dehydration like headache, fatigue, and muscle cramps. The most significant component of sweat is sodium, so sodium is commonly used in sports drinks and hydration supplements, with various other electrolytes like potassium and magnesium blends. But sports drinks aren't the only way to get your electrolytes.

127

Eating your electrolytes

Drinking your daily allowance of fresh water, combined with a diet of hydrating, mineral-rich foods, is a great way to make sure you're getting your daily electrolytes. Plus, food tastes good. Coconut water gets a lot of attention for being one of the most complete single food sources of potassium, magnesium, and sodium—and it's great! However, there are many other mineral-rich food sources that, prepared with a little bit of sea salt, become well-rounded sources of electrolytes.

These mineral-rich foods include:

● **LEAFY GREENS:** High in potassium, magnesium, and calcium.

● **AVOCADOS:** High in potassium, a single avocado contains about 15% of RDV.

● **NUTS AND SEEDS:** Excellent sources of magnesium, with around 20–30% of RDV per 1-ounce serving.

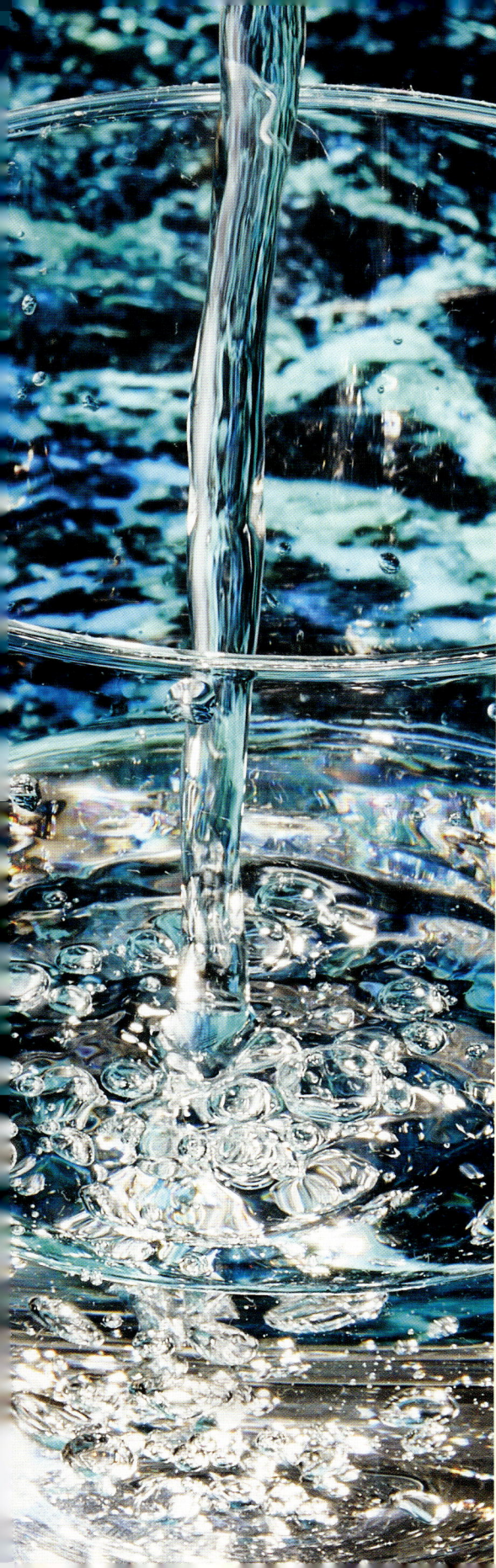

We Need Salt for Hydration

If you stopped ten people on the street and asked whether salt was hydrating or dehydrating, the responses you would get would probably be about 50/50. And in this case, everyone would be right. Sodium is a key electrolyte, essential for hydration, but an excess can disrupt the balance of electrolytes in our body and cause dehydration (as well as many other issues).

It's also important to recognize that not all sodium is created equal. The sodium most of us get in the standard American diet is typically highly refined, processed, and devoid of other trace minerals. Processed foods often contain sodium in concentrated forms for flavor enhancement and preservation. They contain amounts of sodium that are so high you couldn't add that much naturally if you tried!

Avoiding sodium altogether is necessary only if you have a distinct medical reason. We always recommend controlling your salt intake when you can by adding quality sea salt to your food and getting naturally occurring sodium from the foods you're consuming.

Non-processed foods that are naturally high in sodium include:

- Beets and beet greens
- Swiss chard
- Celery
- Seafood
- Seaweed, particularly kombu and dulse

We love to cook using seaweed in broth to add flavor, depth, and high-quality sodium.

Why is sodium important for hydration?

WATER FOLLOWS SODIUM

Water naturally moves toward the area of higher sodium concentration. This movement of water due to the osmotic gradient is what helps maintain proper fluid balance in the body.

WATER RETENTION

Sodium helps the body absorb and retain water. This is why it's often included in electrolyte tablets and rehydration drinks. It is especially effective during intense exercise or when recovering from dehydration due to illness.

FLUID BALANCE

Sodium helps regulate the amount of water in and around cells, maintaining the body's fluid balance. It is crucial for preventing dehydration and ensuring that cells function properly.

ELECTROLYTE BALANCE

Sodium works with other electrolytes like potassium and chloride to conduct electrical impulses in the body, which are vital for muscle contractions and nerve signaling.

The Role of Glucose in Hydration

Glucose is simply sugar, and it plays a significant role in hydration, particularly through its influence on how your body absorbs water and electrolytes.

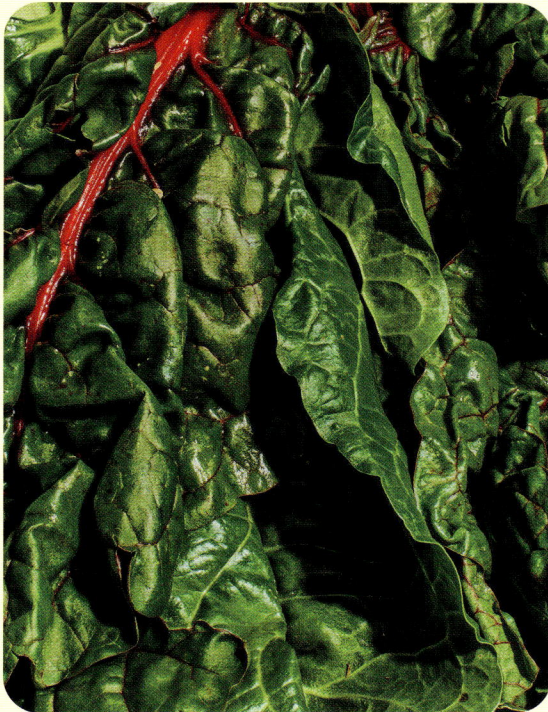

Glucose:

FACILITATES SODIUM AND WATER ABSORPTION

Glucose enhances the absorption of sodium in the small intestine through a process known as the sodium-glucose cotransport mechanism. Sodium absorption, in turn, increases water absorption because water follows sodium.

PROVIDES ENERGY FOR CELLULAR FUNCTION

Glucose is a primary energy source for cells, including those that maintain the fluid balance in your body. Proper hydration ensures that cells can efficiently utilize glucose for energy, which supports overall body functions.

CONTRIBUTES TO OSMOTIC BALANCE

Which is crucial for maintaining the proper distribution of fluids within and outside cells. This balance is essential for normal physiological function and prevents issues like cell swelling or dehydration.

In summary, glucose aids in the efficient absorption of water and electrolytes, supports cellular energy needs, and helps maintain osmotic balance, all of which are vital components of proper hydration.

129

Weighing Your WATER OP

We'll admit that choosing a water filter can be complicated. Many of the "best" filtration systems are super-expensive whole-house commitments that aren't accessible to many people. We hope this section will help you to make sense of the options and decide what's best for you.

R
IONS

TAP
SPRING
PURIFIED
ALKALINE
SPRING
FILTERED
TAP
SPRING
PURIFIED
ALKALINE
SPRING
FILTERED
TAP
SPRING
PURIFIED
ALKALINE
SPRING
FILTERED
TAP
SPRING
PURIFIED
ALKALINE
SPRING
FILTERED
TAP
SPRING
PURIFIED
ALKALINE
SPRING
FILTERED

Weighing Your Water Options

TAP, TAP

The Environmental Working Group (EWG), a nonpartisan, nonprofit organization, recently found polyfluoroalkyl substances, also known as PFAS or "forever chemicals," in tap water systems in twenty cities across the US. This is more than a little disturbing, as PFAS have been linked to health problems including cancer, hormone disruption, immune system suppression, cardiovascular disease, and more. PFAS are everywhere, used in many everyday products, including nonstick cookware and waterproof clothing, and they have ended up in our food and water supply. There is little we can do to completely avoid these chemicals, but we can minimize our exposure by using a water filter to eliminate them from our drinking water.

   In addition to PFAS, the water that comes through your tap contains small quantities of many other harmful substances and impurities, ranging from microbial contaminants like bacteria and viruses, to chemical pollutants such as pesticides, and heavy metals like lead and mercury. To determine the quality of your tap water, we encourage you to check out your local water quality report—the Environmental Protection Agency (EPA) Safe Drinking Water Information System (SDWIS) is one of the best ways—to understand where your water comes from and what's in it. Once you determine which toxins you should be most concerned about, it's time to look for a water filtration system.

PURIFIED WATER

Purification goes a step further, by filtering out all physical contaminants in water in addition to using chemical processes to eliminate viruses, biological contaminants, and minerals that filtration alone does not.

Each of the following purification methods offer unique benefits and can be chosen based on your specific needs.

Distillation
Water is heated until it's converted into steam to remove unwanted particles, and the steam is recondensed into liquid water.

Deionization
A process that removes all mineral salts via ion exchange and replaces dissolved minerals with hydrogen and hydroxide particles.

Ozonation
Involves fusing ozone into water to disinfect it. Most companies that bottle water use ozone gas as a disinfectant instead of chlorine due to its less distinct taste and smell.

absolute 1-micron filtration
Forcing water through filters capable of removing particles that are 1 micron (one-millionth of a meter) in size with a high degree of accuracy. This type of filtration is necessary when very fine filtration is needed to remove microscopic contaminants in types of industrial processing (food, pharmaceuticals, etc.). It is not for home use.

ALKALINE WATER

Some people claim that alkaline water is better than anything you could get from the tap, but the science doesn't back it up. Water is a combination of hydrogen and oxygen, and its pH level ranges from 6.5 to 8.5, depending on how acidic or alkaline it is. A pH of 7 is considered neutral, or balanced between acidic and alkaline. If water is below 7 on the pH scale, it's acidic. If it's higher than 7, it's alkaline. Alkaline water enthusiasts claim its increased hydrogen provides greater hydration than regular water, especially after a hard workout. Other supposed benefits include improved metabolism, increased energy, slowing the process of aging, improved digestion, and reduced bone loss.

   However, there is not much research to support these claims, and the body can keep pH levels on an even keel on its own. The whole job of our kidneys is to act as that natural filtration system, balancing pH levels. Our stomach is also a great equalizer. Your gastric juices—a combination of digestive enzymes and hydrochloric acid—neutralize food and drink. Your stomach will re-calcify alkaline water before it can do anything the health claims promise.[13]

FILTERED WATER

At a minimum, filtered water is a must. The best water filters will remove unwanted taste and odor from tap water and screen out harmful chemicals, bacteria, and microbes. It's important to note that filters do not remove viruses. You will need a water purifier for this. When shopping for a water filter, it's best to look for a system that both filters and purifies.

For individuals concerned about PFAS in their drinking water, the most effective treatment methods include granular activated carbon (GAC) filters, ion exchange, and reverse osmosis systems. However, some of these solutions can be costly and complex.

Below are the most common water filtration options to help establish which is the best choice for you:

Pitcher Filters

Pitcher filters are an excellent choice for those seeking a simple, convenient, cost-effective way to improve their drinking water quality. They are easy to use and require no installation. Pitcher filters effectively reduce common contaminants such as chlorine, sediments, and certain heavy metals, improving the taste and odor of tap water. They are affordable and require minimal maintenance.

→ **Pros:** Convenient, affordable, and portable.

→ **Cons:** Limited capacity and slower filtration rate, which may have limitations depending on your household water consumption. The filtration range is limited, although brand dependent. Most are not effective at removing PFAS, trace pharmaceuticals, or heavy metals.

Countertop Filtration Systems

There is a wide range of options for countertop filtration, some offering very high-quality and extensive filtration, and some more limited. Countertop filtration is a great option because it is generally easy to set up and portable.

→ **Pros:** Accessibility, affordability, ease of use, higher water output than pitcher filters, high-quality filtration options

→ **Cons:** Takes up counter space, low flow rate, water waste (depending on unit type). Wide range of efficacy.

Under-Sink Filters

Water filters come in all sizes, shapes, and efficacy, but nothing compares to the under-sink filter. Under-sink filters are effective because they control quality before the water comes out of the tap. When shopping for filters, screen for how many particulates an under-sink option filters out, look specifically for a reverse osmosis system (which filters and purifies), and understand how much water is wasted. It's also vital that your filtration system has been independently tested and certified according to NSF (National Sanitation Foundation /ANSI (American National Standards Insti-

tute) or IAPMO (International Association of Plumbing and Mechanical Officials) standards.

→ **Pros:** Improved water quality, advanced filtration technology options, long-lasting filters, high water capacity

→ **Cons:** Installation complexity, maintenance, potential for leaks, not portable (nor suitable for frequent moves), up-front cost of installation can be high. Range of filtration varies greatly.

Reverse Osmosis (RO) Systems

RO systems are the ultimate filtration system, offering maximum contaminant reduction and purification. They provide the most comprehensive protection against even the most difficult-to-filter substances. The one downside of RO systems is that they typically strip beneficial minerals like calcium, magnesium, potassium, and sodium from water in the process, which is not a huge deal, since we absorb most of our minerals through food. If you want to remineralize your water, though, you can add a pinch of Himalayan salt to it, which adds back minerals like calcium, magnesium, potassium, sodium, phosphorus, and others.

→ **Pros:** Comprehensive, multistage filtration; safety and quality assurance certifications; cost-effective long-term

→ **Cons:** High up-front cost, installation complexity, frequent maintenance, water waste, mineral removal

133

SPRING WATER

About 50 percent of bottled water comes in the form of spring water. The rest is refined tap water. Groundwater, which exists underground in an aquifer, is the source of spring water. It's generally considered pre-purified, as it has traveled through natural filters like limestone, sandstone, and clay to the earth's surface.[14] High-quality spring water is rich in magnesium, potassium, calcium, sodium, and other trace minerals, which are instrumental in filling nutritional gaps in our bodies.[15] Spring water also oxygenates the body's cells, fueling the metabolic processes in the body.

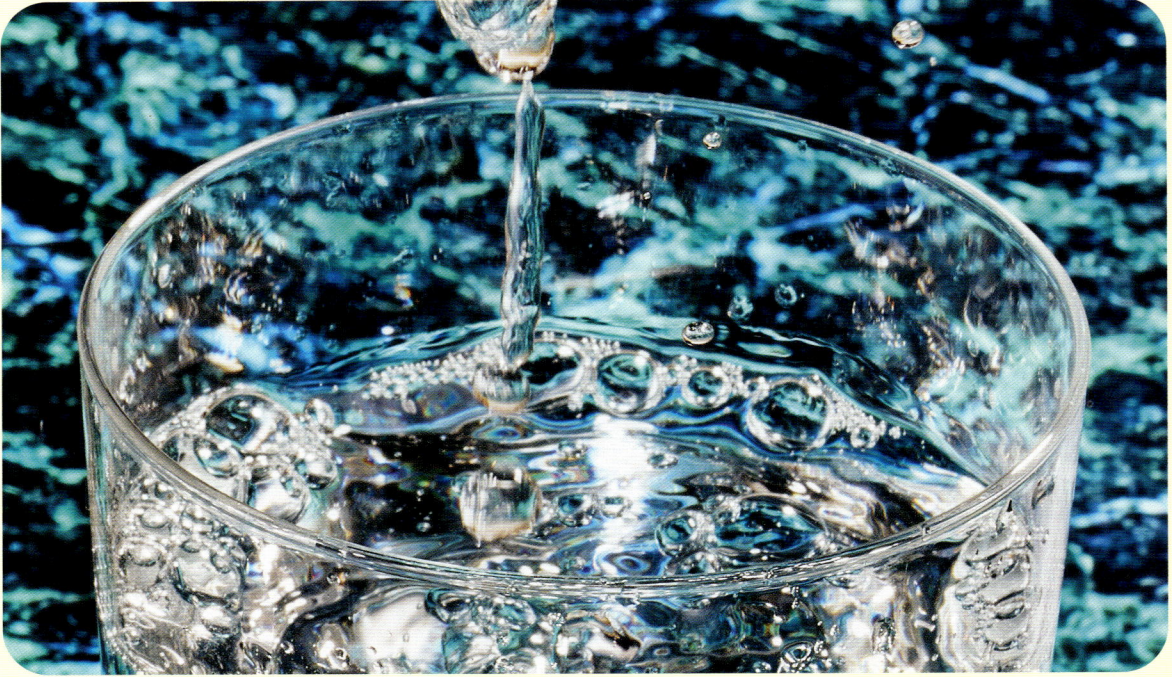

SPARKLING WATER

"The truth is, I've been drinking a bottle of Gerolsteiner water a day for close to twenty years. I'm not exactly sure how or when I decided this would be my thing, but it's hands down my favorite water."
—MEREDITH

When we talk about sparkling water, we prefer sparkling mineral water—not carbonated purified water. Mineral waters will typically be labeled as "mineral water" or "sparkling mineral water," and carbonated water is labeled as "sparkling water" or "seltzer." The difference is the quality of the base water. While purified and carbonated water is fine to drink, the water is usually sourced from nonspecific municipal supplies without the minerals found in natural sources and may feel less hydrating. Mineral water comes from a natural underground source and contains a mineral profile typically listed on the label. While both types count toward liquid intake, the quality of hydration from sparkling mineral water is superior, so that is the only type we would drink to replace pure water.

FLAVORED WATERS

Here's the thing about flavored water: If it gets you to drink more water and you're sipping on it instead of drinking soda, sugary drinks, cocktails, or other high-sugar beverages, it's great. But it isn't going to replace high-quality filtered water because it mostly lacks the natural mineral content to provide deep replenishment. There are now so many carbonated drinks with "natural flavors" (which has a wide range of meanings) on the market that we can't keep up. While we're all for having fun with them, and some of them genuinely taste great, we'd still consider them somewhat of a novelty item.

Let's Talk Water Bottles

Your water quality is also affected by the vessel you're drinking from. Either your water bottle can leach harmful contaminants into your water, or it can be an inert vessel to simply carry water. We prefer the latter. Ultimately, we recommend using glass or metal vessels over plastic, and we'll explain why.

→ **PLASTIC**

Most reusable plastic water bottles are manufactured from plastic polymers such as polypropylene and copolyester, which makes them light and durable. And many of them are also advertised as free of the chemical bisphenol A (BPA), commonly used in plastics until recent studies linked it to hormonal disruptions in humans. Most plastic water bottles do not use BPA. The problem is that they've replaced it with bisphenol S, which we have limited information on. Until more research has been done on these alternatives, we recommend sticking to glass and metal over plastic. If you are using a plastic water bottle, we suggest handwashing over washing in a high-heat dishwasher, which increases the chance of chemical leaching.

→ **METAL**

Most metal water bottles are made from stainless steel or aluminum. Metal eliminates concerns about chemical leaching that we have with plastic. We recommend metal water bottles that aren't lined with plastic, epoxy, or resin, which some manufacturers add to mask the tin-like taste caused by metal vessels.

→ **GLASS**

Glass is our number-one choice of material for a reusable water bottle. Glass is made of natural materials and is inert, so there is no danger of chemicals leaching into liquids when heated or cooled. Glass also doesn't hold flavor—some people complain that water in plastic or metal bottles tastes like chemicals or tin. Glass tends to be heavier than metal or plastic and slightly less functional for that reason. Fortunately, there are now many glass water bottles that are sold with exterior cushioning to make them a more practical option.

How Much to Drink, and When

Slow and Steady Wins

Many of us have gotten away from a common-sense approach to all forms of consumption, and drinking water is no exception. There is little to no benefit to waking up and "chugging" (as is often recommended) a ton of water. Your body needs time to absorb the water you're drinking. Consuming massive amounts of water quickly can overwhelm your kidneys, dilute electrolytes, and disrupt the fluid balance in your body, essentially doing more harm than good. Plus, drinking water too quickly can be uncomfortable.

To ensure proper hydration and absorption, we recommend drinking gradually throughout the day. We also like to minimize water intake after 5 p.m. so we aren't up all night peeing.

Drinking with Meals

We've all been to restaurants where they constantly refill your glass with ice water, and sometimes, on a hot day, this is what we want. But keep in mind that when we drink large amounts of water with meals, we dilute digestive enzymes that work to break down our food and help us digest. This is why we recommend drinking most of your water separate from meals, and during a meal, that you only sip it lightly. Most resources indicate that drinking small amounts of water with meals does not seem to negatively impact digestive enzymes and certainly helps you pace your meal and enjoy the food.

Water-Rich Foods First

We prefer to eat water-rich foods at the start of a meal in a practice called "food combining." Food combining involves consuming foods in a particular order to aid digestion. Common principles of food combining include eating fruits alone, not mixing proteins with carbohydrates, and consuming fats separately from other food groups. While we do not follow these rules strictly, we do recommend trying to eat fruits (specifically the watery ones) alone and seeing if you notice an improvement in how you feel. Food combining is not backed by science, but many other cultures have methods of food combining that are largely ignored in the West, and we believe that there is something to it.

"On my honeymoon in Bali, I met a shaman who told me I had been dehydrated my whole life. He said that if I didn't change something, my organs would eventually stop functioning well. I'd never loved the taste of plain water and had a hard time getting myself to drink it (I needed to use better filtration!). So, I had some work to do to get myself drinking enough water throughout the day. The following is my routine for drinking more water and ensuring that it gets absorbed."

—KAT

KAT'S ROUTINE

● **7:00**AM
I wake up and drink one glass of room-temperature water with lemon.

● **8:00**AM
I fill a gallon-size jug with filtered water, so that I can begin to track my water intake. I try to drink 2 gallons of water gradually throughout the day, separate from meals.

● **12:00**PM
I eat a hydrating lunch. I am all about eating water-rich foods. I usually opt for a crunchy salad, or beet carpaccio to keep it interesting.

● **7:00**PM
I stop drinking and eating liquids for deeper sleep.

MEREDITH'S ROUTINE

● **7:00**AM
I try to drink at least 16 ounces of water first thing in the morning. More than that and I feel like I'm forcing myself to drink it.

● **8:00**AM
If I remember, I put my water in a liter container so that I can gauge the amount I drink throughout the day. I'm not obsessive about the amount I drink. I try to listen to my body's thirst signals. If I've worked out it's easy to drink. If I haven't, I might not be as thirsty. I like to drink out of a mason jar because it is a simple and effective way of measuring the amount.

● **12:00**PM
If I've been consistent with sipping throughout the morning, on a typical day I will have consumed around 50 ounces of water by lunchtime.

● **2:00**PM
After two o'clock I'm typically drinking green tea or a Gerolsteiner sparkling water and have mostly moved away from flat water.

● **5:00**PM
If I take a hot bath, I will always have water and something "fun" to sip on, whether that's a N/A cocktail, an occasional glass of wine, or sparkling water with lemon. I do try to wind down the volume of liquid consumed after five o'clock, so I don't have to pee in the middle of the night.

● **8:00**PM
I keep a glass of water by my bed out of habit from my childhood. I can't sleep without it even though I barely drink it.

137

CONCLUSION

Water is life, the fuel and source of energy, vitality, and good health. While the quality of the water we drink is important, eating vibrant foods filled with natural water and juices is the best way to hydrate at a cellular level. So much emphasis is placed on *drinking* water, but we want to inspire you to eat your water too! Let's get started with some nourishing, hydrating recipes.

138

The Recipes

→ "Suero" Mineral Drink

→ Boneless Mineral Broth

→ Cauliflower Tabbouleh

→ Zucchini Pasta

"Suero" Mineral Drink

We've already touched on the importance of minerals in hydration, and this recipe is here to say: If you're not making your own electrolyte drink, we highly recommend trying. Not only does it taste great, but we think you'll find it more refreshing.

SERVES 1

—————————

12 ounces (360 ml) cold mineral water (we love Gerolsteiner)

1 teaspoon sea salt

Juice of 1 lime

Lime slice, for garnish

140

How to make?

Stir the water, sea salt, and lime, then garnish and sip.

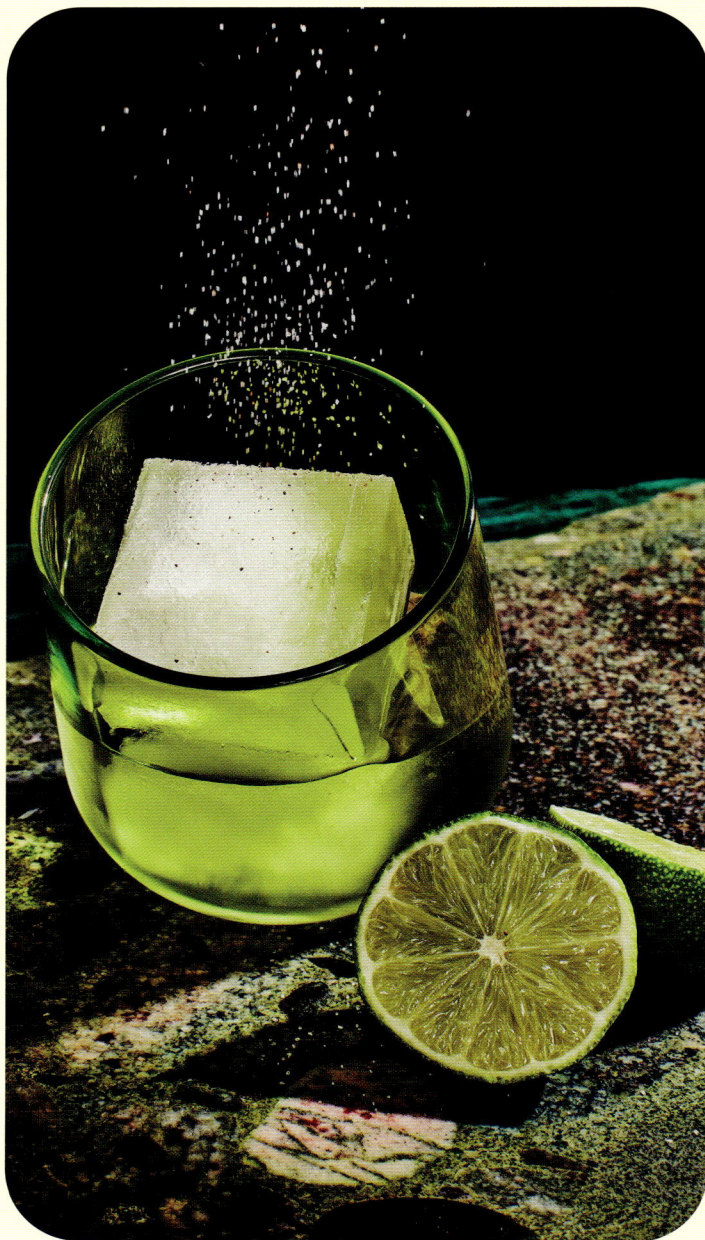

Boneless Mineral Broth

MAKE ABOUT 8 CUPS (2 L)

2 to 3 tablespoons (30 to 45 ml) olive oil (or you can use water to soften the veggies)

2 medium carrots, chopped

3 stalks celery, chopped

1 leek (white and light green parts), chopped

2 to 3 cloves garlic, minced

1-inch (2.5 cm) piece fresh ginger, peeled and grated

1 cup (35 g) assorted dried mushrooms (or just shiitakes)

2 tablespoons tamari (optional)

4 to 5 pieces dried kombu seaweed (2 to 3 inches / 5 to 7.5 cm each)

1 handful dried wakame seaweed flakes

1 handful dulse seaweed flakes

1 bunch fresh parsley, including stems

1 bunch kale, stems removed (optional)

2 teaspoons sea salt or to taste

2 teaspoons cayenne (optional, to taste)

We've all heard the hype around bone broth, and while some of the claims are substantiated, others are not. What makes bone broth such a big deal is the mineral density. Our vegan version is rich in calcium, magnesium, potassium, and iron—all of which make up the building blocks to collagen, bone density, and cellular hydration. We love to sip this on its own, or use it as a base for soups and stews. If your seaweed is whole, tear or cut it into 2- to 3-inch (5 to 7.5 cm) pieces.

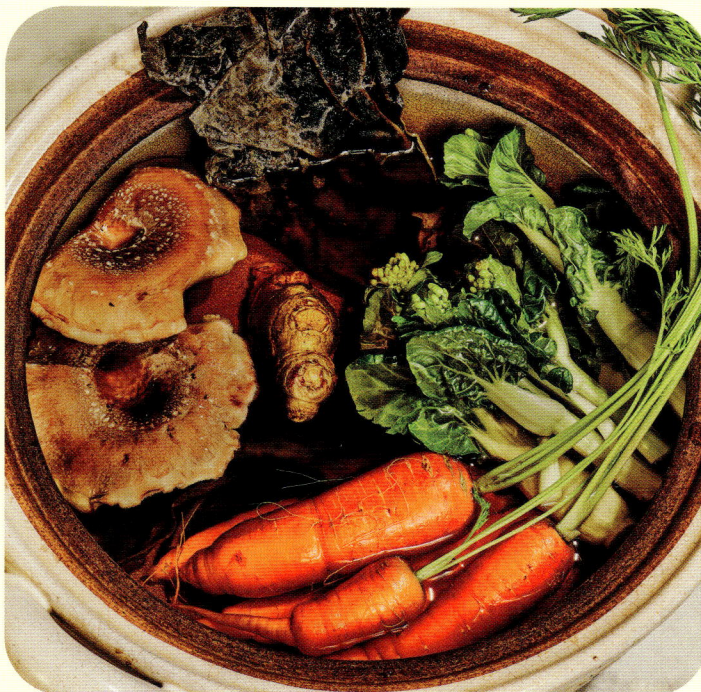

How to make?

In a large pot, heat the olive oil over medium-high heat. Add the carrots, celery, leek, garlic, and ginger and sauté for 7 to 10 minutes, until the vegetables are soft and the aromatics release their scent.

Add the mushrooms and tamari, if using, and cook for a few minutes, until the mushrooms start to soften, then add the kombu, wakame, dulse, parsley, and kale, if using.

Pour in 8 to 10 cups (2 L to 2.4 L) filtered water, or enough to cover the vegetables and seaweed. Add the sea salt and cayenne, if using.

Simmer for at least 45 minutes or up to 6 hours. The longer you cook the broth, the more flavor is extracted.

Remove or thinly slice the kombu before serving. You can store the broth in the refrigerator for up to 5 days, or freeze.

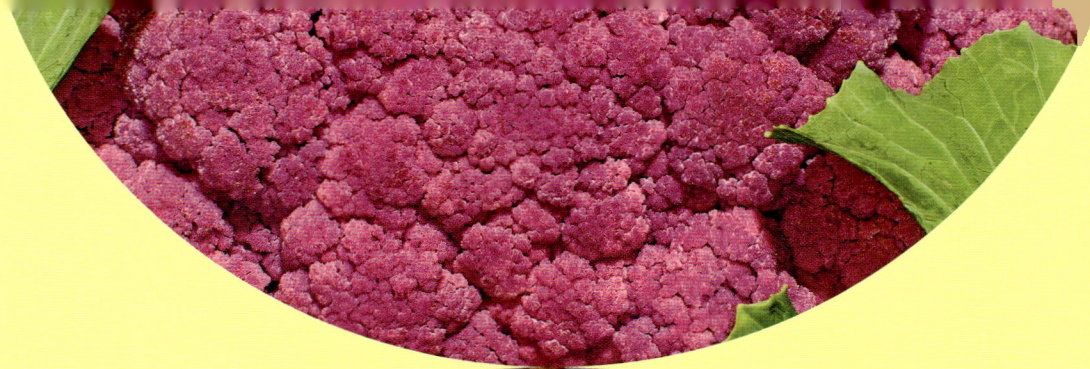

142

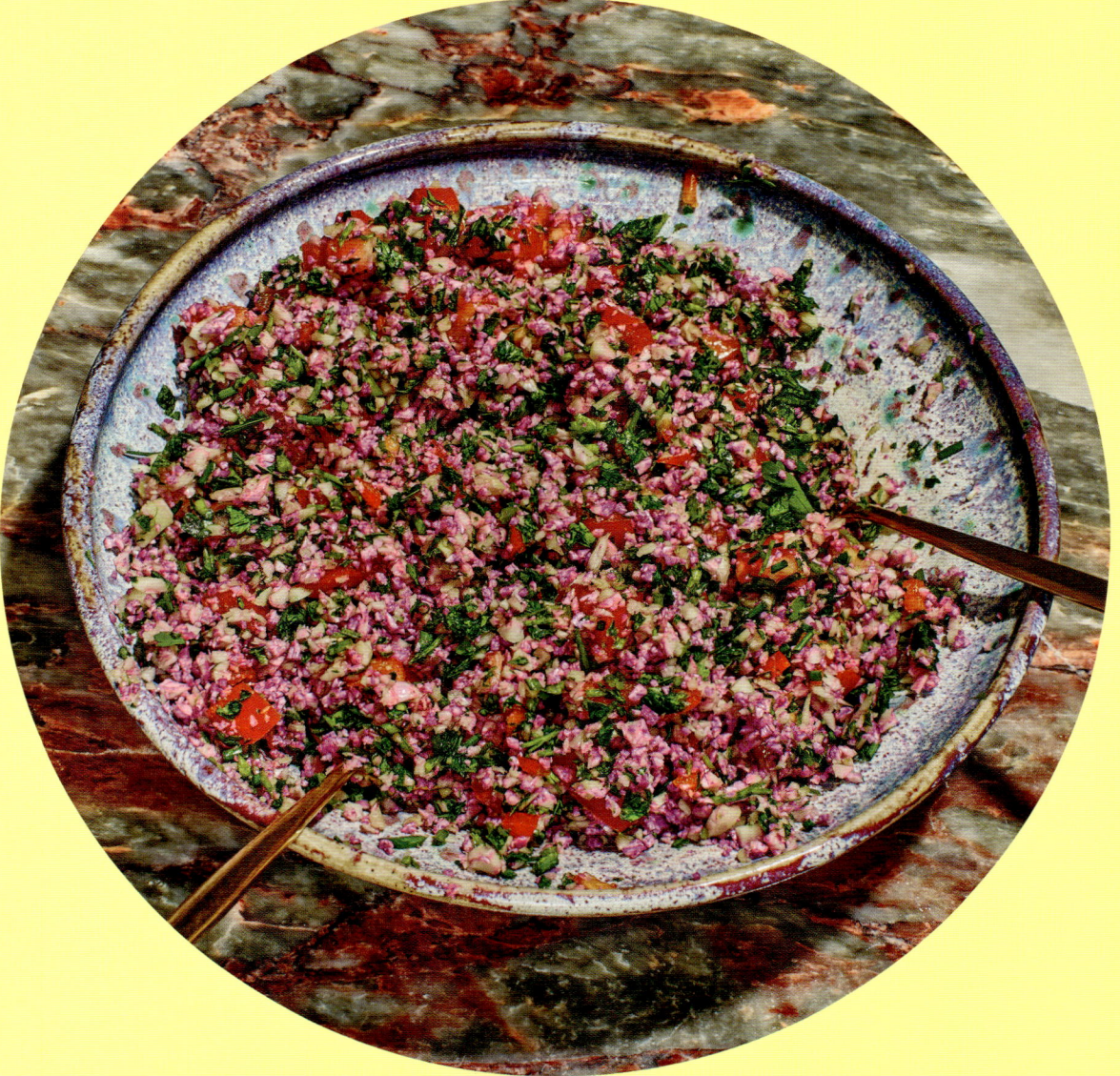

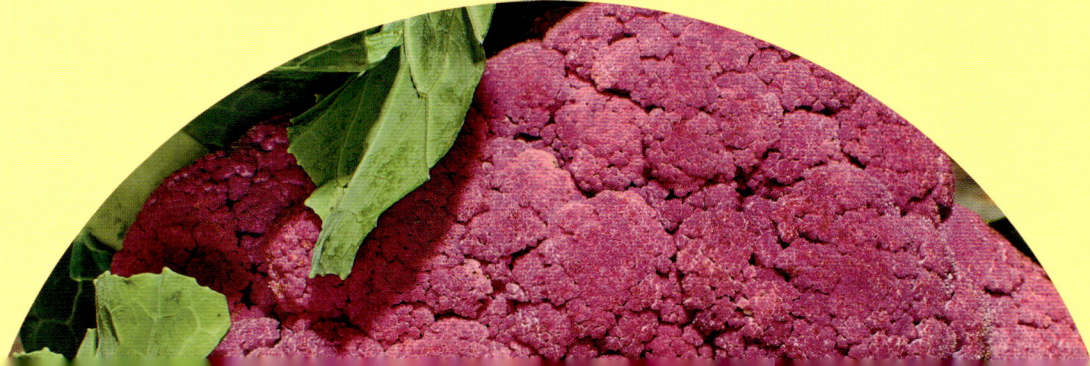

Cauliflower Tabbouleh

When thinking about the recipes to include in this book, Kat and I unanimously agreed that Cauliflower Tabbouleh had to live here. Not that we have anything against bulgur, but the cauliflower version is one of those swaps that is equally as good as the traditional one and easier to make. The raw veg content is high-density, packed full of hydrating vitamins and minerals.

SERVES 4 OR 6
AS A SIDE

---

1 medium head cauliflower (20 to 25 ounces / 550 to 700 g)

1 cup (145 g) cherry tomatoes, halved

1 medium cucumber, diced

½ cup (25 g) finely chopped chives

1 cup (50 g) finely chopped fresh parsley

½ cup (25 g) finely chopped fresh mint leaves

½ cup (75 g) raisins, chopped

½ cup (65 g) pine nuts, chopped (optional)

Juice of 2 lemons

¼ cup (60 ml) extra-virgin olive oil

1 teaspoon sea salt or more to taste

½ teaspoon black pepper or more to taste

How to make?

Remove and discard the leaves and stems from the cauliflower. Grate the cauliflower using a box grater or run the florets through the food processor with the grating attachment. (If you have the patience, finely chop it yourself.)

In a large bowl, combine the cauliflower, cherry tomatoes, cucumber, chives, parsley, mint, raisins, and pine nuts, if desired.

Toss with the lemon juice, olive oil, sea salt, and pepper.

Let marinate for at least 30 minutes before serving.

143

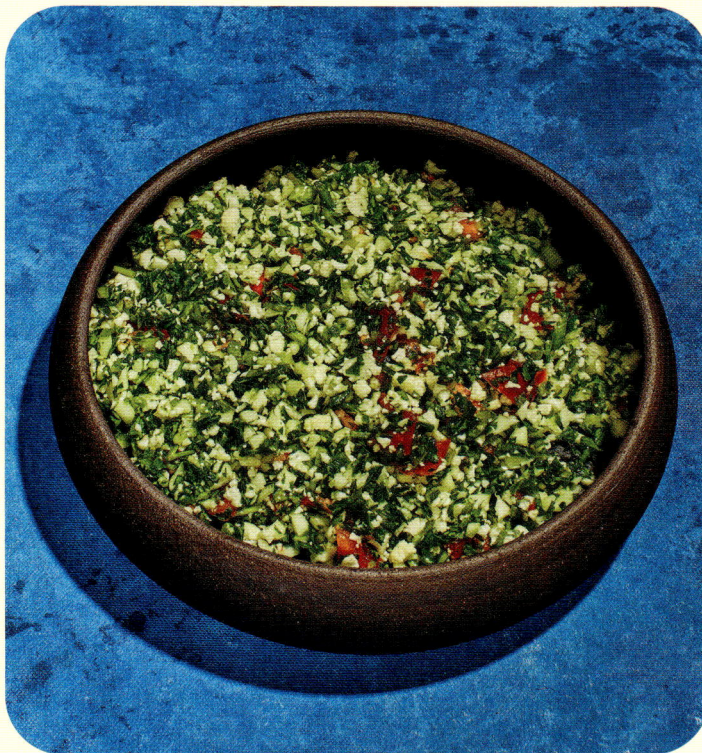

Lentil and Tempeh Bolognese over Zucchini Pasta

This dish was a turning point for me when it came to feeding my family. It's a proper hearty, healthy dish that everyone (including my seven-year-old) enjoyed. I love using a spiral slicer to make vegetable noodles. This is a kitchen gadget that can be purchased for around $30, but some stores sell spiralized noodles presliced in the produce section. If you don't own a spiral slicer, you can make vegetable noodles on a mandoline, using the julienne blade. If neither of these is an option, feel free to use your favorite pasta.

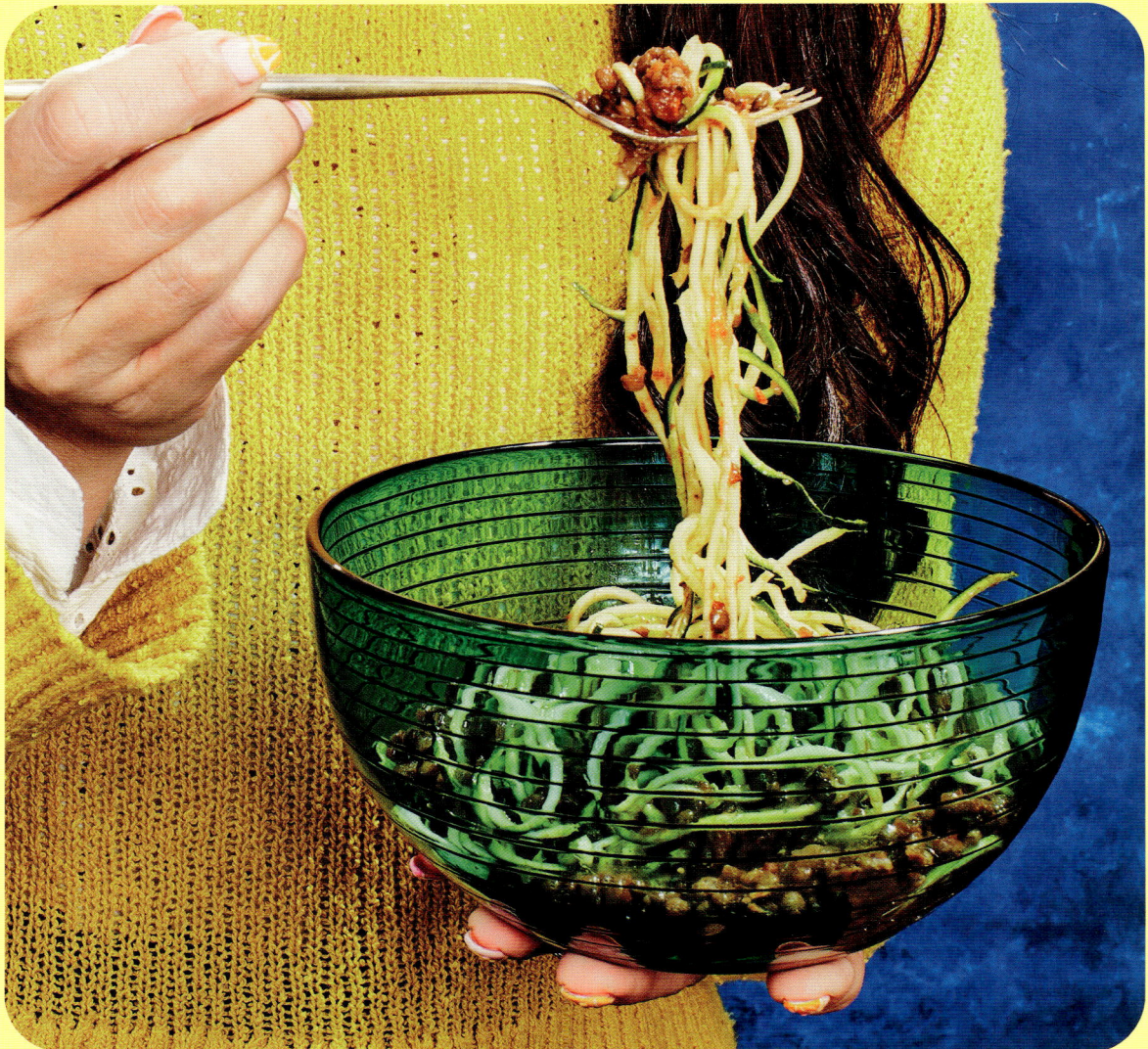

---

1 tablespoon olive oil

1 large onion, finely chopped

2 cloves garlic, minced

2 medium carrots, finely chopped

2 stalks celery, finely chopped (optional)

1 cup (190 g) dry green or brown lentils, rinsed

1 (8-ounce/225-g) package tempeh, chopped (optional)

1 (28-ounce/840-ml) can crushed tomatoes

2 tablespoons tomato paste

1 teaspoon dried oregano

½ teaspoon dried thyme

½ teaspoon smoked paprika

1 teaspoon sea salt

¼ teaspoon red pepper flakes (optional)

2½ cups (600 ml) vegetable broth or water

Salt and freshly ground black pepper

About 7 ounces (200 g) spiralized zucchini, or your favorite cooked pasta, for serving

Fresh basil, for garnish

How to make?

Heat the olive oil in a large pot or Dutch oven over medium heat. Add the onion, garlic, carrots, and celery (if using). Sauté until all the vegetables are soft, 7 to 10 minutes, stirring occasionally.

Add the lentils and chopped tempeh (if using) to the pot and stir to combine with the vegetables. Stir in the crushed tomatoes, tomato paste, oregano, thyme, smoked paprika, sea salt, and red pepper flakes (if using). Pour in the broth, add the salt and pepper, and stir well.

Bring to a gentle simmer, then reduce the heat, cover, and cook until the lentils are tender and the sauce thickens, 30 to 40 minutes, depending on how fresh your lentils are.

Remove the lid and cook for about 5 minutes before serving. Add more broth to the sauce if necessary to achieve your preferred consistency.

To serve, plate over spiralized zucchini or your favorite pasta noodles. Garnish with fresh basil and serve.

→ Tip

This Bolognese sauce will last in the refrigerator for up to 4 days, so double the recipe if you'd like! The leftovers are excellent.

145

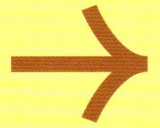

Sleep

So Good

We need sleep. It's essential to our mental and physical health.

And yet, the average adult is chronically sleep deprived, contributing to a growing health crisis in our modern world. Why aren't we sleeping enough? For starters, as a culture, we seem to have decided that chronic sleep deprivation indicates strength or productivity. Factors like stress, health issues, and our constant use of devices are also contributing to our poor sleep quality. Misconceptions about sleep abound. What most of us don't understand is that insufficient sleep can lead to long-term health consequences that are much more serious than just being tired all the time.

Like the huge gaps in nutrition education, sleep education is a subject barely taught in medical school. According to the Harvard Medical School Division of Sleep Medicine, the number of people suffering from sleep issues will double in the next twenty years; and yet, a survey of most medical school curriculums reveals an average of only two hours or less is spent on formal sleep education within a four-year course. That's barely any time at all! This is significant because sleep disorders can impact virtually every other aspect of our health, from our stress levels to our weight to our digestive health.

"I feel relatively unique when I say that my whole house gets enough sleep. I am blessed to have a child who enjoys sleep as much as my husband and I do, and none of us have an issue making it a priority. Instead of getting worse, my sleep has gotten better with age. I also prioritize and look forward to it. The sleep schedule is nonnegotiable, and I enjoy every minute."

—MEREDITH

What Is Sleep?

Sleep is an essential biological function that leaves our bodies and brains recharged.[1] Sleep is crucial to our health for several reasons, including brain function, immunity, growth and healing, learning and memory consolidation, and emotional regulation. When and how long we sleep—aka our sleep cycle—is regulated by a complex interplay of factors that include our hormones, biology, genetics, environment, and lifestyle.

Sleep regulation

Our sleep is regulated by our circadian rhythms, twenty-four-hour cycles that are part of the body's internal clock. In addition to sleep regulation, our circadian rhythms manage body temperature, immune response, hormones, metabolism, and cognitive function. Circadian rhythms are controlled by "biological clocks" located in organs and tissues throughout the body[2] that are all synced up with a "master clock" called the suprachiasmatic nucleus (SCN), located in the brain's hypothalamus. The presence and absence of sunlight have the biggest influence over our circadian rhythms, in addition to food intake, stress, physical activity, social environment, and temperature.

If we don't sleep when our body tells us that it's time to, or if we sleep for long periods during the day, our circadian rhythms can get thrown off. There are many reasons why this might occur, including travel across time zones, shift work, stress, or a noisy and/or bright sleep environment. When this misalignment occurs, it's important to act, because it can wreak havoc on our overall health.

Sleep stages

Healthy sleep occurs in a cycle that repeats multiple times over the course of a night and that is divided into two distinct phases: rapid eye movement (REM) sleep and non-rapid eye movement (NREM) sleep.

NREM sleep is further broken down into three substages:[3]

→ STAGE 1 (N1)
  The transition between being awake and being asleep

→ STAGE 2 (N2)
  The stage of light sleep before entering deeper sleep

→ Stage 3 (N3)
  Deep sleep, also known as "slow-wave sleep"

Humans cycle through all stages of non-REM and REM sleep several times during the night, with increasingly longer, deeper REM periods occurring toward morning.[4] A "sleep cycle" usually begins with stage 1 of non-REM sleep and continues through stage 2 non-REM, stage 3 non-REM, and REM sleep. A typical night of sleep comprises four to six sleep cycles.

149

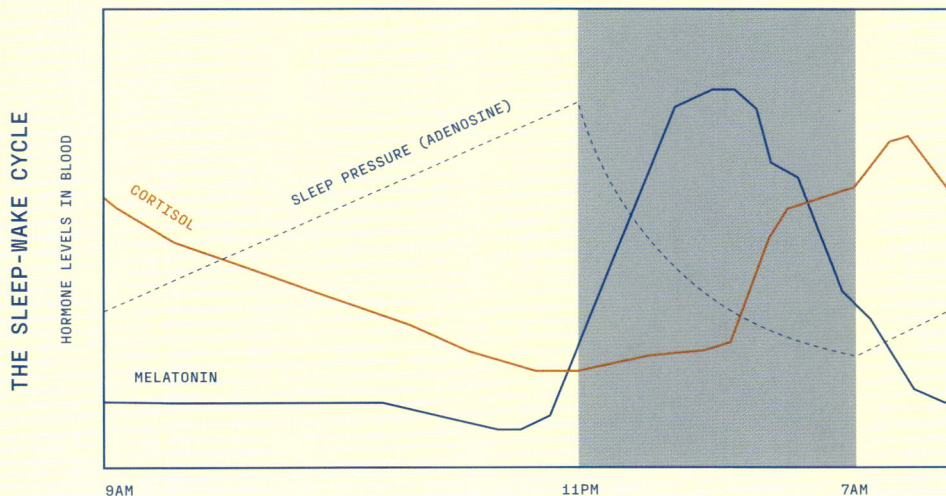

THE SLEEP-WAKE CYCLE

HORMONE LEVELS IN BLOOD

SLEEP PRESSURE (ADENOSINE)

CORTISOL

MELATONIN

9AM   11PM   7AM

During the various stages of sleep, crucial aspects of physical and biological restoration occur. All of them play a significant role in optimizing health and well-being. **These processes include:**

ENERGY RESTORATION

This is the obvious one that we all associate with sleep. This restorative cycle happens by replenishing glycogen (stored glucose) that provides the brain and body energy during waking hours.

BRAIN DETOX AND COGNITIVE FUNCTION

Healthy sleep is vital for cognitive functioning, mood, and mental health.[6] Sleep promotes overall brain health immediately and in the long term through the glymphatic system, which is responsible for clearing out waste from the brain and becoming more active during slow-wave sleep. This system helps to remove toxins and reduces the risk of neurodegenerative diseases. REM sleep is closely linked to cognitive functions, memory consolidation, and learning.

TISSUE REPAIR, GROWTH, AND PHYSICAL RESTORATION

Deep sleep, or slow-wave sleep (stage 3), is essential for the body's regeneration and repair processes. During deep sleep, blood flow increases to the tissues, including muscles, bones, and skin, thus increasing the delivery of essential nutrients and oxygen needed for healing and growth.[7]

HORMONE RELEASE

Sleep regulates hormones like cortisol and melatonin, essential in managing stress and the circadian rhythm. Good sleep regulates stress through hormonal balance, so having one without the other is impossible. Growth hormone is also released during sleep and is vital for childhood development and tissue repair.

IMMUNE FUNCTION

Sleep and the circadian rhythm system help regulate and influence the immune system and its function. Slow-wave sleep especially is vital for optimizing immune functions and forming long-term immunological memory, supported by specific hormonal changes during this sleep stage.[8]

EMOTIONAL WELL-BEING

Sleep is essential to our ability to cope with the stressors of everyday life in an emotionally regulated manner. Disruptions in sleep patterns can impact mood, stress levels, and emotional resilience. Healthy sleep is essential for mood and mental health.[9]

How Much Sleep Do We Need?

The amount of sleep we need per day varies with age and stage of life. The following recommendations come from the American Academy of Sleep Medicine (AASM) and the Sleep Research Society (SRS):[10]

→ INFANTS (4 TO 12 MONTHS): 12 to 16 hours

→ TODDLERS (2 TO 4 YEARS): 11 to 14 hours

→ CHILDREN (5 TO 12 YEARS): 9 to 12 hours

→ TEENAGERS (13 TO 18 YEARS): 8 to 10 hours

→ ADULTS (18 AND OVER): 7 to 9 hours

Do those numbers surprise you? Over time, our sleep patterns have changed, and we are getting less sleep now than at any time in history. Consider:

● In 1959, the average adult age forty to seventy-nine was getting eight hours per night, with less than 15 percent of adults reporting a sleep time of under seven hours a night.[11]

● By 2002, the average sleep time for adults had decreased to seven hours per night, with more than one-third of adults sleeping less than seven hours a night.[12]

● As of 2024, the average amount of sleep for adults in the United States is less than seven hours per night.

It is estimated that 50 to 70 million Americans suffer from sleep disorders, and with so many sleep-deprived adults walking around trying to perform daily tasks, the negative health implications are enormous.

What Are the Consequences of Poor Sleep?

Lack of sleep leaves us more than just tired. Insufficient sleep has been linked with seven of the fifteen leading causes of death in the United States, including cardiovascular disease, cancer, stroke, increased risk of accidents, diabetes, sepsis, and hypertension.[13]

The subject of sleep is poorly covered, even in medical education, with the consequences of many sleep disorders being misinterpreted as other clinical conditions, primarily neurological or psychiatric disorders.[14] We need more sleep, and we need to understand why.

These are a few of the most prominent health implications of lack of sleep:

COGNITIVE FUNCTION

Cognitive function impairment is relatively self-explanatory. If you are feeling exhausted, it will be harder to concentrate. This can also be dangerous, as extreme exhaustion can make you less alert and more accident prone. Lack of sleep also affects the brain's ability to process new information and impairs learning and retention. This is especially important for school-age children who frequently do not get optimal sleep.

RISK OF CARDIOVASCULAR DISEASE

The correlation between sleep and cardiovascular disease is less intuitive, but insufficient sleep is linked to elevated blood pressure, which is a significant risk factor for heart disease and stroke. Chronic sleep deprivation can also contribute to heart disease by increasing inflammation in the blood vessels, leading to arterial plaque buildup.[15]

METABOLIC DISORDERS

Lack of sleep can lead to insulin resistance and impaired glucose metabolism, increasing the risk of type 2 diabetes. Studies have shown that a sleep duration of 6 hours or less, or 9 hours or more (you can have too much), is associated with an increased prevalence of diabetes and impaired glucose tolerance.[16] A study restricting sleep to 4 hours per night for six nights resulted in impaired glucose tolerance

(IGT) in healthy young adults.[17] Poor sleep affects metabolism by increasing inflammation, reducing glucose efficiency, and elevating cortisol levels. It also disrupts hormones that regulate appetite, leading to increased hunger and snacking.

WEAKENED IMMUNE SYSTEM

Insufficient sleep compromises the immune system through various immune impairments. It is shown to contribute to the overproduction of proinflammatory cytokines. This can result in chronic low-grade inflammation associated with multiple health issues, including a weakened immune system and suppressed immune function.

MENTAL HEALTH ISSUES

Sleep deprivation can exacerbate mood disorders like depression and anxiety, making it harder to manage these conditions. Chronic lack of sleep affects mood through altered brain function, neurotransmitter imbalances, hormonal changes, and impaired emotional processing.

HORMONAL IMBALANCE

Sleep is crucial for regulating various hormones, and when our sleep cycles are out of whack or we are sleep deprived, it can throw the following hormones out of balance:

- Somatotropin (growth regulation)
- Melatonin (sleep-wake cycle regulation)
- Cortisol (stress regulation)
- Leptin and ghrelin (appetite regulation)[18]
- Thyroid hormones (metabolism regulation)

151

Sleep Hygiene

"I highly recommend getting excited about your nighttime routine. For me, this has been the key to getting better and sounder sleep than ever before in my life. Yes, I still have an ounce of teenager inside me who wants to rebel against all sleep hygiene recommendations: 'I'll eat late and stay up late if I want!' But I've caved to the healthier rhythm and typically start a wind-down by 7:30 p.m. I've also discovered a delightful routine that includes stretching, some menthol rub on my shoulders, and ice rolling my face. I'm sure my husband wonders what is going on."

—MEREDITH

152

There is a sweet spot for healthy sleep. As we've touched on, seven to nine hours per night is generally considered healthy for most adults. But there's more to it than that. Healthy sleep is not just about the duration; it is also about the quality and regularity of your sleep, influenced by your sleep habits, or what is known as "sleep hygiene."[19]

Our body's rhythms and functions run best on routine, and our sleep cycles are no different. Although good sleep hygiene can look a little different for each person, there are a few science-backed rules that we consistently adhere to:

Maximize exposure to natural light during the day. Aim to get exposure to natural sunlight during the day, especially in the morning. We recommend that you step outside and get a dose of natural sunlight as soon as possible after waking. This can simply be stepping outside and taking a few deep breaths before turning your face to the phone, having a cup of coffee on the porch if you are able, or taking a short walk. Watching the sunset is equally beneficial in helping to regulate your circadian rhythm, as the natural light of the sunset can signal to your body that it is time to wind down. Both sunrise and sunset are transitional periods in the day and can encourage mindfulness and promote a feeling of relaxation, leading to sounder sleep.[20]

Limit exposure to artificial light and electronics at night. It is essential to minimize exposure to blue light from screens in the evening. Blue light during the day suppresses melatonin production, but exposure before bed (when you want an increase in melatonin) can disrupt normal circadian rhythms.[21] Ideally, we recommend putting your devices away one to two hours before bed (if one hour is more realistic, that is OK). If you must use your device in the evening, consider using blue light–blocking glasses or screen filters to reduce the impact of artificial light on your sleep. Ultimately, we believe being mindful of how you use devices in the evening is almost as important as the choice whether to use them.

"It's hard to practice what we preach on this one, as watching a show in bed to relax at the end of the day is one of my favorite things to do. My personal approach is just about being mindful. I feel like scrolling and mindless searching is so much worse for your sleep then relaxing and watching a show even though they both emit blue light."

—MEREDITH

Eat within an optimal metabolic window. The sophisticated rhythm of hormones dictating our sleep also regulates our metabolic processes. Eating at inappropriate times (when our bodies are less ready for food) promotes metabolic risks by disrupting sleep patterns, altering the circadian rhythm, and impairing melatonin production, all of which negatively affects our sleep quality. The secondary effects of these disturbances cause many issues, including excessive weight gain, increasing cortisol levels, and disrupting our digestion. For example, leptin, a hormone that regulates appetite and energy balance, drops off significantly after 7 p.m. When we eat after that 7 p.m. window, things shift, our melatonin production can be affected, and the cascade of negative side effects begins.[22]

Experiment with time-restricted eating by limiting your food intake to a specific window during the day that feels good for you and works for your schedule. This approach can help regulate your body's internal clock and improve sleep quality.

Engage in regular exercise. Regular exercise helps regulate melatonin production. Incorporate regular physical activity into your daily routine, but be mindful of the timing of vigorous exercise. A hard workout done too close to bedtime can be overstimulating, interfering with sleep and delaying melatonin production. Instead, aim to exercise at least three to four hours before bed to reap the sleep-promoting benefits without the side effects of increased stimulation. Gentle yoga, walks, and things of that nature are typically fine closer to bedtime and may promote better and deeper sleep.

Optimize your sleep environment. Creating a sleep environment that works for your sleep routine can be one of the most enjoyable aspects of sleep hygiene. We recommend a dark, quiet, and calming atmosphere as optimal for sleep. Use blackout curtains, earplugs, or a white noise machine to minimize disruptions and promote better sleep quality.

Establish a bedtime routine. Develop a relaxing pre-sleep routine to signal to your body that it's time to wind down. Make sure that this routine is one that you will enjoy and look forward to. If you use a wearable device to track sleep, it is interesting to gauge which behaviors impact sleep quality most, as it can be slightly different for everyone. Engage in calming activities such as reading, listening to soothing music, or practicing mindfulness before bedtime.

Limit caffeine and alcohol consumption. This one probably goes without saying, but be mindful of your intake of caffeine and alcohol, especially in the hours leading up to bedtime. Both substances can disrupt sleep patterns and impair sleep quality, so it's best to consume them in moderation or avoid them close to bedtime. Caffeine works by blocking the action of adenosine, a neurotransmitter that promotes sleep, reducing our feelings of tiredness and making it harder to fall asleep. Caffeine is also metabolized differently among individuals. For some people, caffeine can linger in the body for up to eight hours or more. This prolonged presence can delay the onset of sleep and reduce sleep quality, even if consumed earlier in the day. Alcohol disrupts your sleep in various ways but primarily by disrupting sleep patterns. As alcohol is metabolized, it can wake you up throughout the night (including the need for frequent urination). It disrupts time spent in the REM stage of sleep, leading to less-restorative sleep patterns.

Many experts recommend limiting alcohol consumption to one drink per day and avoiding alcohol for at least three hours before bed for better sleep. Others suggest that any amount of alcohol during the day, regardless of the time, will disrupt sleep patterns.

Manage stress with breathing exercises. Incorporate breathing exercises, such as diaphragmatic or box breathing, to help calm your mind and body before bedtime. Deep, slow breathing can activate the parasympathetic nervous system, promoting relaxation and better sleep.

153

Science-Backed Ways to Improve Your Sleep

Sleep supplementation involves using specific nutrients and compounds to support and enhance sleep quality. Common supplements include melatonin, which regulates the sleep-wake cycle, and magnesium, known for its role in promoting relaxation by calming the nervous system. Other supplements like L-theanine and valerian root can reduce stress and anxiety, facilitating easier sleep onset. The science behind these supplements is rooted in their ability to influence neurotransmitters like GABA and serotonin, which play critical roles in relaxation and sleep regulation. However, it's essential to note that sleep supplements should complement, not replace, healthy sleep habits.

154

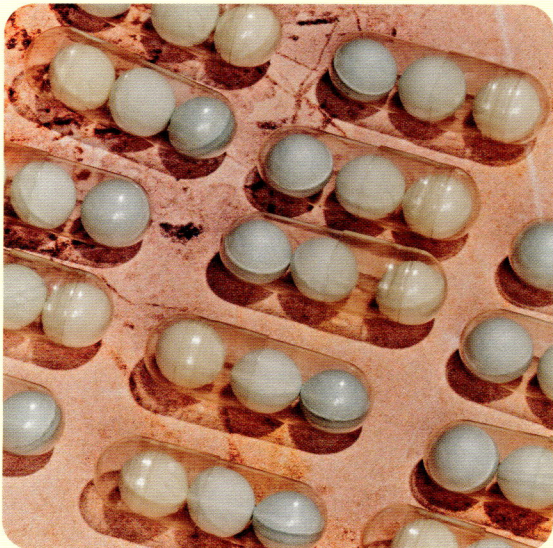

Melatonin

The most popular scientifically backed sleep supplement is melatonin. Melatonin is a hormone naturally produced by the body and secreted by the pineal gland in the brain.[23] Melatonin is vital to our circadian rhythm, involved in signaling "time of day" and "time of year" to our bodies. Melatonin also works effectively as a dietary supplement, and is available as both a prescription and over-the-counter sleep aid.[24]

Melatonin production and release are stimulated by darkness and inhibited by light. Melatonin production can be disrupted by bright light from natural sources like the sun and by shining light from artificial sources like lightbulbs, TV screens, and smartphones. Melatonin's secretion increases soon after it begins to get dark, reaches a peak between 2 and 4 a.m., and gradually decreases during the second half of the night.[25]

Our body's melatonin production varies with age. Newborns produce very little melatonin. Melatonin production increases in early childhood, peaks around puberty, and then declines in adolescence. It is interesting to note that for teens melatonin is released later in the evening, which makes them less tired at night, but their sleep needs are still high, which is often a mismatch with school schedules. Melatonin production continues to decrease gradually throughout the lifespan, which may contribute to the decreased sleep quality commonly experienced by older adults.[26]

Risks of Taking Melatonin Supplements

Melatonin supplements can benefit short-term sleep issues, but they carry potential risks and side effects, especially with long-term use or high doses.

These risks include:

● DAYTIME DROWSINESS: Taking too much or too late can cause drowsiness the next day.

● HORMONAL EFFECTS: Long-term use can interfere with hormone levels and potentially impact puberty in children.

● MOOD CHANGES: Some users report feelings of depression or mood swings.

● MEDICATION INTERACTIONS: Can interact with blood thinners, immunosuppressants, diabetes medications, and birth control pills.

● DIGESTIVE ISSUES: Nausea, cramping, and diarrhea are common side effects.

● HEADACHES AND DIZZINESS: These symptoms can occur, particularly with higher doses.

● SLEEP CYCLE DISRUPTION: Improper use can disrupt your natural sleep cycle.

How to Take Melatonin Properly

Melatonin supplements can help regulate sleep patterns when used correctly. Timing, delivery method, and avoiding interactions are all important considerations.

● TIMING: Take melatonin at least thirty minutes before you plan to go to bed. This allows enough time for the supplement to start working. Always take melatonin at the same time in the evening to help regulate your sleep cycle.

● DELIVERY METHOD: Pills and tablets are the most common and easy-to-use supplements, available in various dosages. Sublingual tablets dissolve under the tongue for faster absorption. Liquid melatonin allows for more precise dosing and faster absorption.

● AVOID INTERACTIONS: Avoid consuming alcohol or caffeine when taking melatonin as these substances can alter its effectiveness. Consult a healthcare provider to ensure melatonin does not interact with any other medications that you may be taking.

● ONLY USE SHORT-TERM: Melatonin is generally recommended and best for short-term use, such as adjusting to a new time zone or dealing with temporary sleep disruptions. If you rely on melatonin for an extended period, consult a health care provider to identify and address underlying sleep issues.

Magnesium

Magnesium plays a critical role in numerous bodily functions, including muscle and nerve function, blood glucose control, and blood pressure regulation, making it important for both physical and mental health—and an effective sleep aid. It supports energy production and improves sleep quality by regulating neurotransmitters and hormones (like cortisol) that calm the nervous system.

For sleep, some of the best forms of magnesium include:

● MAGNESIUM GLYCINATE: This is often considered the top choice for sleep because of its high bioavailability and calming effects. Glycine, an amino acid, has its own sedative qualities, which can help promote relaxation and improve sleep quality without causing digestive upset.

● MAGNESIUM BISGLYCINATE: This is a highly bioavailable form of magnesium, chelated with glycine to enhance absorption and reduce the likelihood of digestive discomfort. It is often used to support muscle relaxation, sleep quality, and nervous system health.

● MAGNESIUM THREONATE: This form is known for its ability to cross the blood-brain barrier, making it effective for cognitive support and nervous system relaxation.

● MAGNESIUM CITRATE: Magnesium citrate is often used for its mild laxative effect, but it also promotes relaxation and can be beneficial for sleep. People with sensitive digestion may want to use it in smaller amounts or combine it with other types.

● MAGNESIUM TAURATE: This form combines magnesium with taurine, an amino acid also known for its calming effects on the nervous system. Magnesium taurate is thought to promote restful sleep without gastrointestinal side effects.

We recommend finding a magnesium supplement that includes a diverse variety of magnesium sources to have the most high-quality impact. Ideally it would include at least three of the above.

155

What's the Deal with Wearables?

"I'll admit that I was skeptical about sleep wearables, mostly because sleep has never been a big issue for me. I figured I didn't need one. However, when I experimented with using one for a month, the data was super exciting and told me a lot about what is best for the quality of my sleep."

—MEREDITH

156

Sleep wearable devices are gaining popularity and attention as an effective way to monitor and learn about our sleep patterns and quality. These gadgets range from smartwatches and fitness trackers to dedicated sleep monitors worn on your wrist, finger, or mattress.

Even if you don't have trouble sleeping, we recommend giving wearables a shot to learn about your own sleep patterns.

These are a few reasons we recommend them:

• Wearables track sleep patterns and provide valuable information about your health. By analyzing your sleep (even temporarily), you can start to identify patterns and behaviors that affect your sleep quality and make informed changes to improve them.

• Health management through early detection: Sleep wearables monitor heart rate and breathing patterns, which can be helpful in the early detection of potential health issues.

• Motivation and goal setting: If you need accountability toward healthier habits, sleep wearables are an excellent tool for monitoring progress and tracking goals.

• Wearables are convenient and easily integrated with daily routines. They are a step toward self-improvement, with minimal effort required.

We predict sleep wearables will become even more popular over the next five years as people prioritize sleep and recognize the value in sleep quality. Technologies like these are simple and effective ways to learn more about your personal health. We think they are an essential part of the modern wellness toolkit.

MEREDITH'S ROUTINE

"I'm a good sleeper, and I always have been—even with sleep habits that used to include staying up too late, drinking too much, and sometimes eating dinner at 10 p.m. As anyone who has worked in restaurants knows, that life is not conducive to good sleep habits. These days, my routine looks different, and I look forward to getting into bed every night."

—MEREDITH

● 6:30^{AM}

Wake naturally. If I'm getting high-quality sleep, I will wake naturally by 6:30, which is when I normally set an alarm.

● 7:15^{AM}

When I can, I step outside for natural light and take a deep breath while drinking my Americano.

● 2:00^{PM} (TEATIME)

I love the pick-me-up of green tea after lunch. The caffeine in green tea releases more slowly than coffee, and the combination of caffeine plus L-theanine makes me feel less jittery. This will always be the last caffeine I have each day.

● 5:00–6:00^{PM} (WIND DOWN)

This is when I'll have a wind-down drink. I love the nonalcoholic cocktail alternatives that include active ingredients like tart cherry, passionflower, L-theanine, and sometimes hemp.

● 8:30^{PM} (READ OR WATCH SOMETHING)

Although we know it's important to eliminate blue light, my husband and I really do enjoy watching a show together to relax. If you feel like this disrupts your sleep or you usually stay up late, then eliminate it. If you get to bed at a reasonable hour and enjoy watching TV beforehand, I believe it's OK.

"With three kids, getting quality sleep is something that I strive for above all else. If I don't get good sleep, I can't be my best for them, and I can't focus on my work. I also end up eating unhealthily and doing things I regret. Once I learned about sleep hygiene and how to prioritize my space and rituals around sleep, my whole life changed."

—KAT

158

● **6:30**^{AM}

Wake up, preferably naturally (but sometimes it requires an alarm).

● **7:00**^{AM} (NATURAL LIGHT EXPOSURE)

I step outside first thing in the morning instead of checking my phone right away. This can help with your sleep cycle later in the day, even if it's just a short walk outside and doing a quick stretch.

● **10:00**^{AM}

Sometimes I will enjoy a matcha as a midmorning pick-me-up.

● **12:00**^{PM} (STOP CAFFEINE)

This is easier on some days than others, but limiting caffeine intake to the morning hours can be hugely beneficial.

● **5:00**^{PM} (SEE THE SUNSET)

I've been experimenting with getting natural light in the evening; if you can catch the sunset, even better.

● **6:00**^{PM} (TRANSITION TO EVENING)

I change my clothes to a nighttime wind-down wardrobe to indicate that I am shifting from daytime duties and into a more relaxed state.

● **6:30**^{PM} (WIND-DOWN MOCKTAIL)

I limit alcohol consumption and recommend not drinking at least three hours before bedtime. I love a nightcap consisting of herbs and adaptogens and our go-to tart cherry drink.

● **7:00**^{PM} (DINNER ENDS)

I stop eating as early as possible to limit my melatonin production and allow my body to rest. This is also an excellent time to stop drinking liquids.

● **8:00**^{PM} (TURN DOWN THE LIGHTS)

This is the time I try to put away devices and screens and eliminate as much artificial light as possible from the house.

● **8:30**^{PM} (SELF-MASSAGE OR RED-LIGHT THERAPY)

This is an excellent time to massage my face or use tools like a red-light mask for ultimate relaxation.

● **9:00**^{PM} (TAKE MAGNESIUM OR MELATONIN)

An hour before bedtime is the ideal time to take a sleep aid like magnesium or melatonin.

We're not the only ones who get excited about getting a good night's sleep.

Once you experience how much better you feel with high-quality sleep, it is undeniable how important it is. We hope you've taken away an understanding from this chapter that good sleep isn't just about avoiding that groggy, tired feeling—although, of course, it is that too. Sleep is much more foundational to our overall health than was previously understood and is a major player in keeping our whole system in check. Sleep gives our brains a chance to clear out toxins and sort out memories—it helps repair tissues, boost the immune system, and even regulate hormones.

Plus, it feels good.

Have no fear; the following recipes will not make you sleepy. They are simply inspired by the ingredients known to help you ease into the evening and promote a healthy night's sleep.

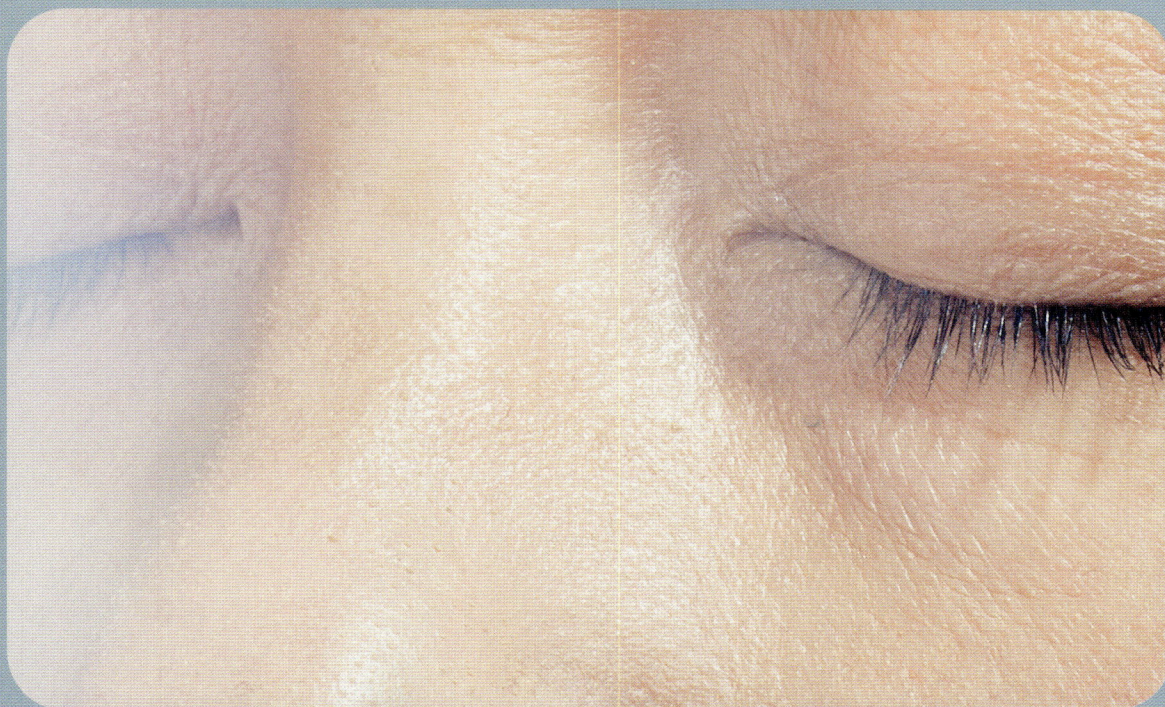

The Recipes

→ **Tart Cherry Nighttime Elixir**

→ **Spicy Walnut Meat and Herbs on Crispy Rice Paper**

→ **Green Coconut Stew with Turmeric Tofu**

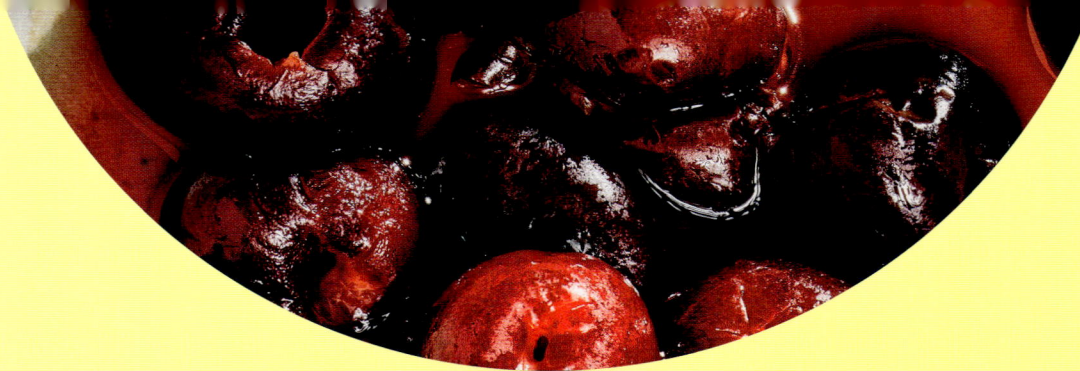

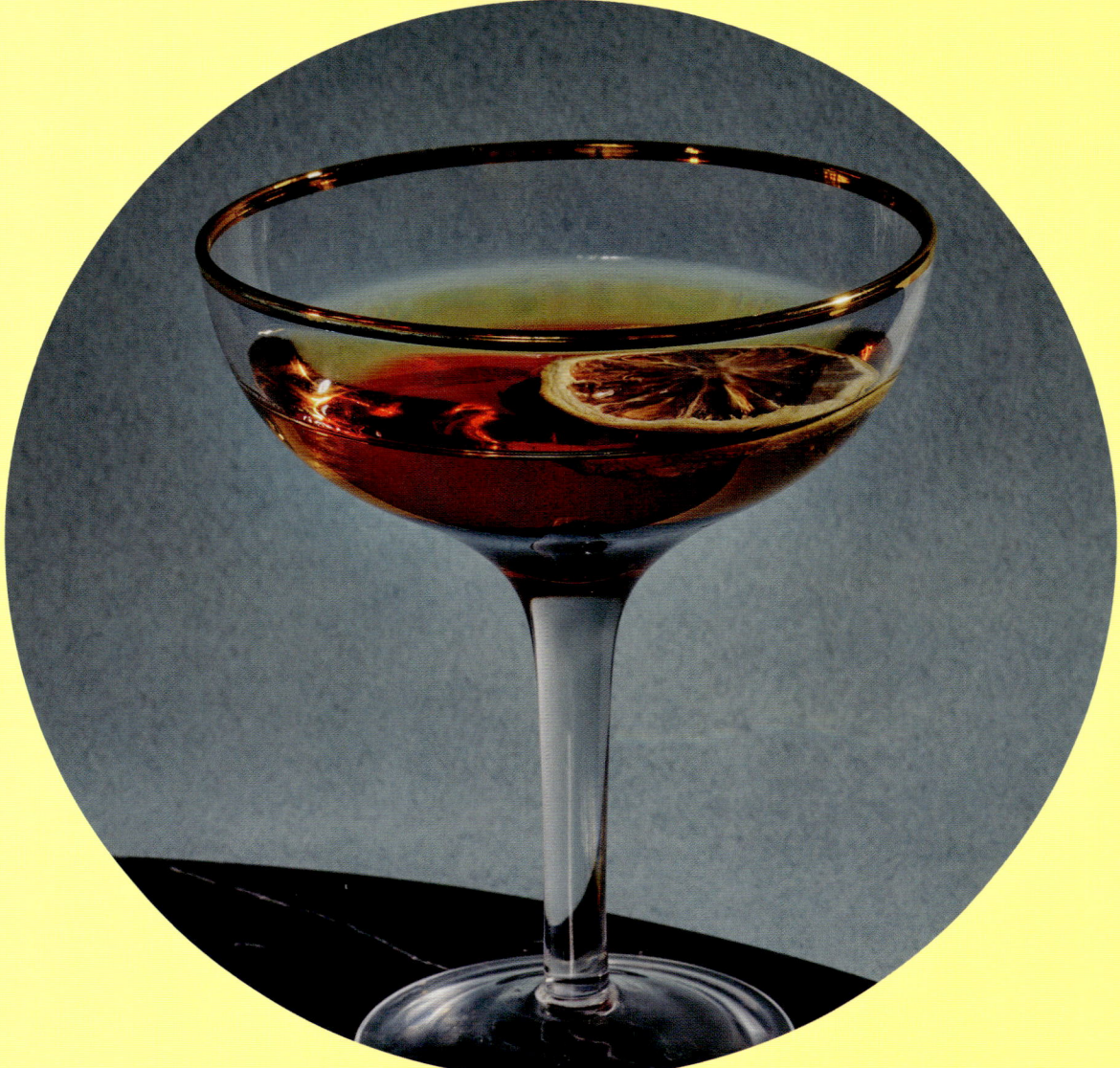

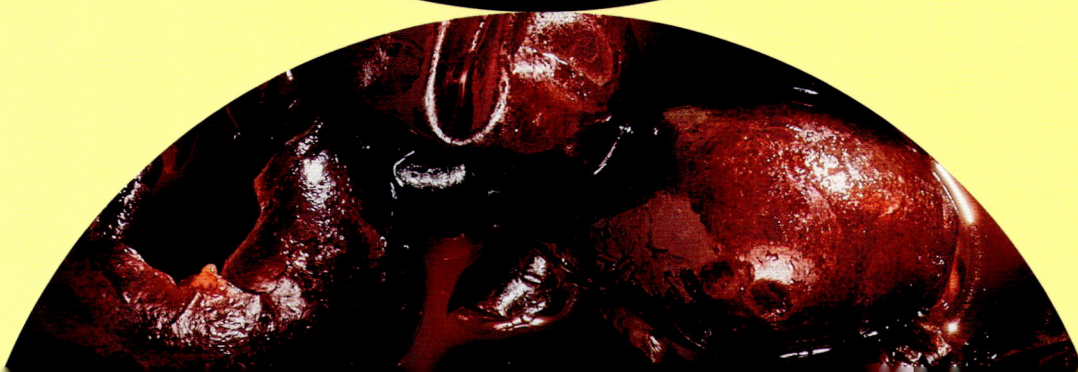

Tart Cherry Nighttime Elixir

MAKES 2 DRINKS

½ cup (120 ml) tart cherry juice

½ cup (120 ml) white or red verjus

½ cup (120 ml) hibiscus tea or herbal tea of your choice

1 teaspoon honey

Ice (optional)

How to make?

Shake the cherry juice, verjus, tea, honey, and ice (if using) in a cocktail shaker, strain, and serve.

If you prefer it warm, omit the ice and add the tea while it's still hot.

Stir before serving.

We absolutely love wine and really value what we call a "transitional" beverage—something that takes you from the energy of the day to nighttime. We've become obsessed with making functional at-home mocktails, and this is one of our favorites. Tart cherry juice is one of nature's best sources of melatonin.

Use white verjus for lighter flavor, red for a richer, bolder drink. Shake with ice for a chilled cocktail, or serve this elixir warm or at room temperature to help ensure sweet dreams.

163

Spicy Walnut Meat and Herbs on Crispy Rice Paper

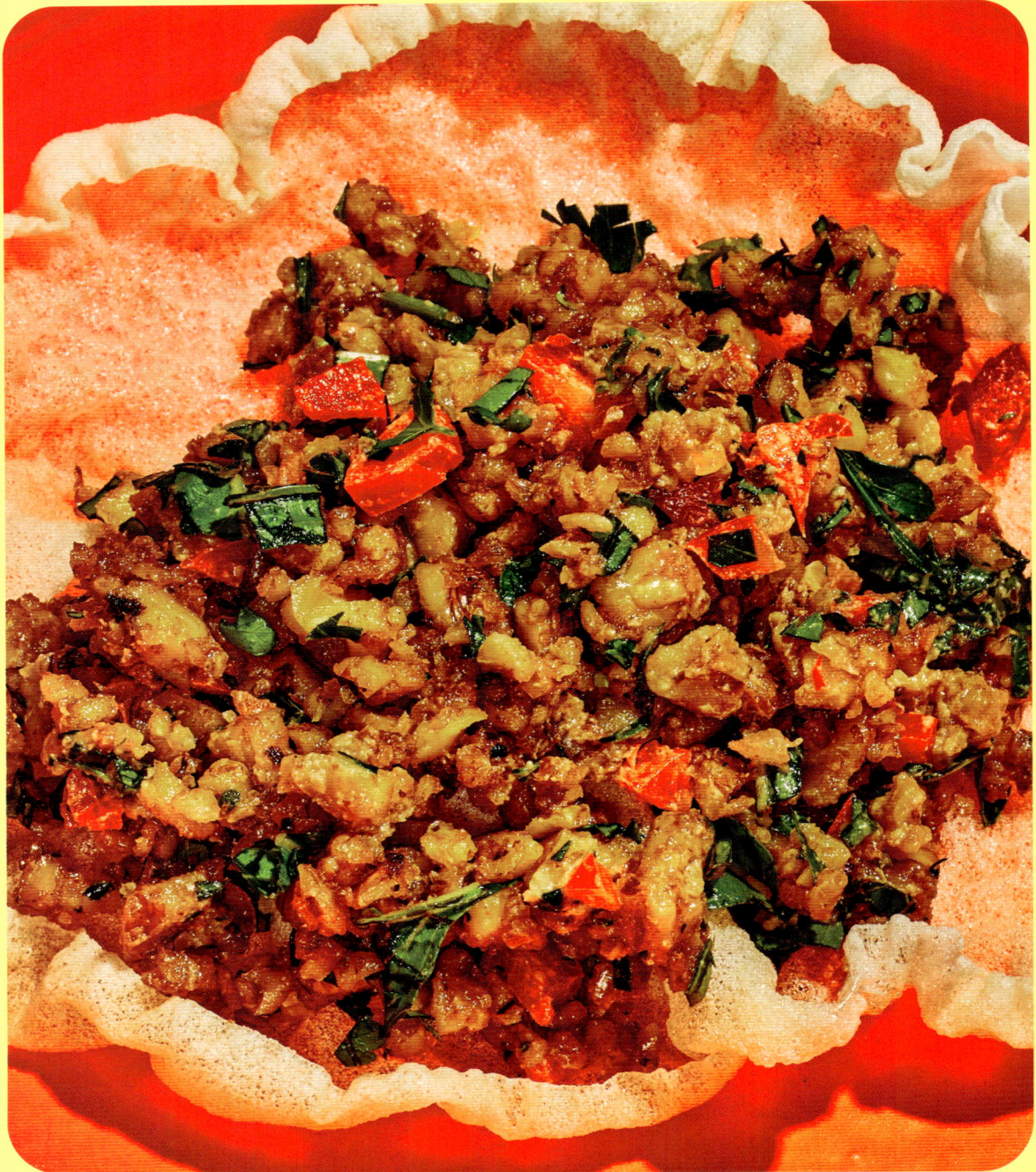

FOR THE SPICY WALNUT "MEAT" FILLING

2 cups (190 g) walnut halves or pieces

1 tablespoon tamari or soy sauce

1 clove garlic, minced

1 tablespoon vegan fish sauce (optional)

1 tablespoon fresh lemon juice

1 tablespoon sesame oil

1 teaspoon ground cumin

1 teaspoon ground coriander

½ teaspoon chili powder or to taste

Pinch salt, or to taste

1 red pepper, finely chopped

½ cup (25 g) chopped fresh mint leaves

½ cup (20 g) chopped fresh cilantro

½ cup (25 g) chopped fresh parsley

2 to 3 green onions, thinly sliced

1 to 2 red chile peppers, finely chopped (optional, for extra heat)

FOR SERVING:

8 to 12 sheets rice paper or 8 to 10 butter lettuce or cabbage leaves

1 cup (240 ml) avocado or rice oil, for frying the rice paper

Sesame seeds, for garnish

Lime wedges

How to make?

→ Make the walnut meat

In a food processor, pulse the walnuts until they reach a crumbly texture (do not overprocess). If you don't have a food processor you can pulse in a blender or finely chop.

Add the soy sauce, garlic, fish sauce, lemon juice, sesame oil, cumin, coriander, and chili powder and pulse just until well combined. You want the mixture to be loose.

Taste and adjust for salt and chili powder.

→ Finish the filling

Put the walnut meat in a medium bowl. Add the red pepper, mint leaves, cilantro, parsley, green onions, and chile peppers (if using) and toss to distribute evenly.

→ Prepare the crispy rice paper

Heat about 1 inch (2.5 cm) oil in a medium saucepan to about 350°F (175°C). You want to make sure the pan is large enough to fit the rice paper wrappers.

Using tongs, drop one sheet of rice paper in the oil at a time and watch it crisp up almost immediately. Remove with tongs to a paper towel to remove excess oil.

Use immediately or store in an air-tight container; these will stay crisp for about 3 days.

→ Assemble and serve

Serve the crispy rice paper (or lettuce or cabbage leaves) alongside the walnut meat filling, sesame seeds, and lime wedges and let everyone assemble their own appetizers.

165

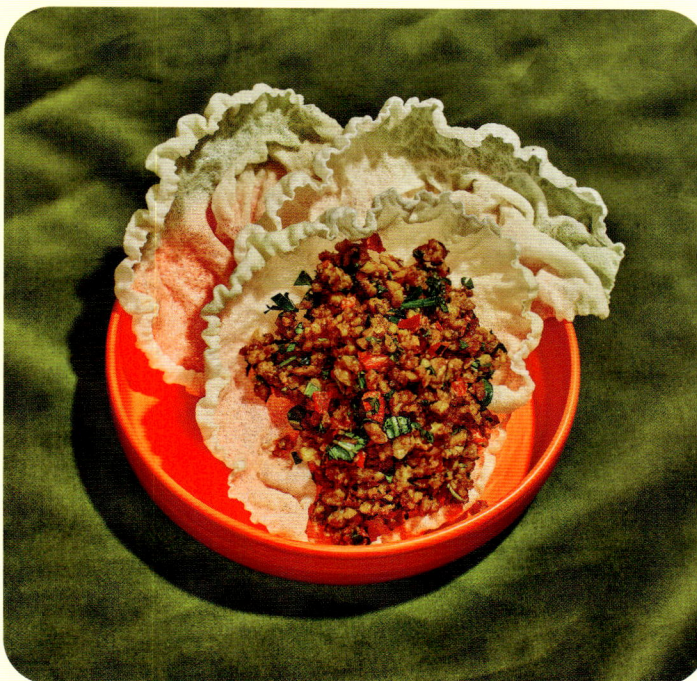

Green Coconut Stew with Turmeric Tofu

SERVES 2 TO 4

FOR THE TOFU:

1 pound (455 g) extra-firm tofu, patted dry and cut into 1-inch (2.5 cm) cubes

1 teaspoon turmeric powder

1 teaspoon garlic powder

FOR THE GREEN COCONUT STEW:

2 tablespoons coconut oil or olive oil, plus more for sautéing the tofu

1 teaspoon cumin seeds

1 large onion, finely chopped

1 tablespoon grated fresh ginger

1 tablespoon grated garlic

2 green chile peppers, finely chopped

1 teaspoon turmeric powder

1 teaspoon ground coriander

1 teaspoon garam masala

1 pound (455 g) fresh spinach, washed and chopped, or 1 (16-ounce) bag frozen chopped spinach

1 can (13.5 ounces / 405 ml) coconut milk

Pinch of sea salt

How to make?

In a medium bowl, toss the tofu with the turmeric and garlic powder and set aside.

Heat the 2 tablespoons coconut oil in a large pan over medium heat. Add the cumin seeds and toast for 1 minute, then add the onions and sauté for 5 to 7 minutes, until they are soft and lightly golden brown.

Add the ginger, garlic, chiles, turmeric, coriander, and garam masala to the onions and give it a stir to create a highly fragrant base. You can add a little water at this point, just enough so that the spices don't stick to the bottom of the pan.

Add the spinach, and cook until the greens are tender and wilted, 3 to 5 minutes. Pour in the coconut milk and bring to a simmer to thicken.

Depending on what style you prefer, you can leave the curry as is or turn it into a smooth green sauce. Remove it from the heat and puree the curry in a high-speed blender or using an immersion blender. Return to the pan and keep warm while you prepare the tofu.

In a skillet over medium-high heat, fry the tofu in a little oil until golden on all sides, about 5 minutes. Using a spatula, remove the tofu to a plate.

To serve, ladle the stew into bowls and top with the tofu.

"I make this recipe most frequently out of anything in my arsenal. My daughter calls it 'tofu with green sauce,' and every time she asks for it, it's music to my ears. If you always keep a can of coconut milk and a bag of frozen spinach on hand, this becomes an easy, last-minute go-to for weeknight meals served over rice or other grains. I like to mix in other greens like collards or kale; it's a good use for greens that might be a little past their prime."

—MEREDITH

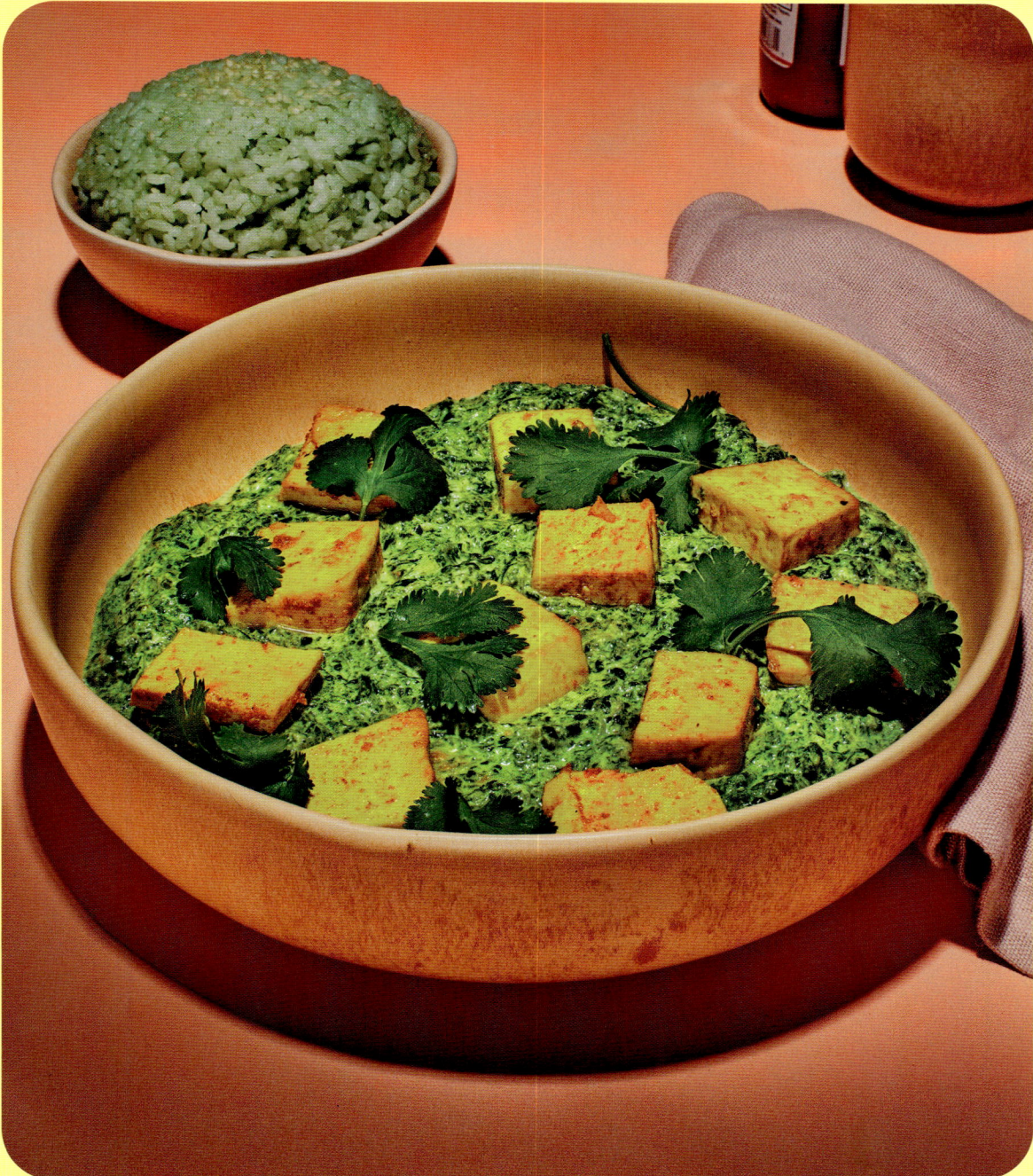

Help

Your

Self

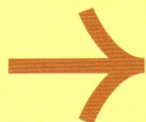

"High stress has always been my default mode. I saw a therapist from ages twenty to thirty, and it helped me to understand how to better deal with my anxiety. When I was younger, I didn't experience the physical manifestations of stress that I do now; it only affected how I felt. But as I've gotten older, I've noticed that when I'm not effectively managing my stress, it shows up in various physical health symptoms, including skin conditions and body pain. When these symptoms creep up, it's an excellent reminder to me that I need to get ahead of my stress and get back to my morning routine, supplements, and daily breath practice."

—KAT

Chapter 6

"My stress levels have for sure increased with age. Some of this is hormonal, and some of it I attribute to the responsibilities of "adulting." Between career, finances, relationships, and parenting, there is so much to juggle. I notice my stress creeping up with obsessive thinking patterns and an inability to focus. For years, I thought that my exercise routines were about physical fitness. It was only recently that I had a lightbulb moment where I recognized that exercise is my most effective tool for stress management. I like to think of exercise as a cortisol detox."

—MEREDITH

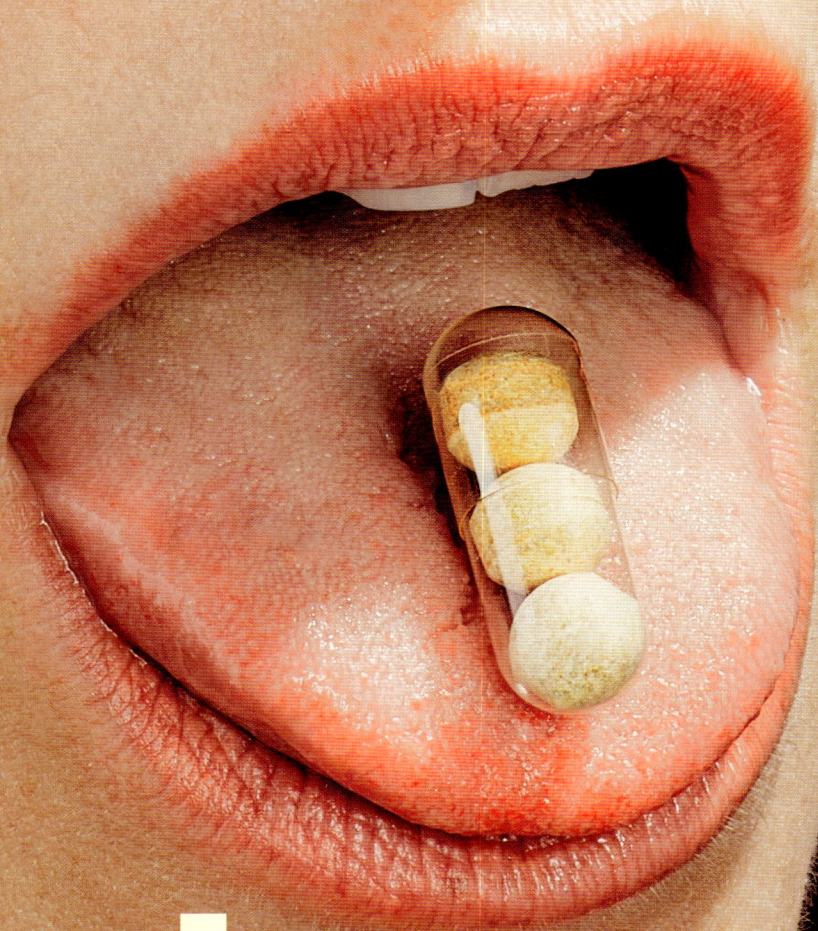

Stress

Less

Stress is a part of our lives. It's impossible to avoid entirely, and we shouldn't want to.

Stress management is one of the top concerns in personal health and workplace wellness. There is good stress, bad stress, traumatic stress, and everything in between. A certain amount of stress is beneficial. However, if not appropriately managed, stress can become chronic, overwhelming us and affecting everything from our physical health to our relationships.

Many times, we misunderstand behaviors that are signs of unmanaged stress: digestive issues, increased heart rate, poor-quality sleep, depressive thoughts, irritability, suppressed immune system. These can all be signs of chronic stress, but when we experience them, we tend to go looking for solutions in all the wrong places. As we discussed in the Introduction, the topics covered in the chapters of this book are interrelated. If you aren't properly hydrated, it will impact your gut health; if you are having gut issues, you may have issues coping with stress. This is just one example of the cyclical nature of the body's systems and how they affect one another.

One of the main misconceptions about stress is that it is entirely environmental or circumstantial.

While external factors play a huge role in our stress levels, learning the tools to cope effectively with stress and improve our response to it can be life-changing.

What Is Stress?

The National Institutes of Health (NIH) defines stress as "a physical and emotional reaction people experience as they encounter challenges in life."[1] Stress is a natural human response, and some forms of stress can be beneficial, which we'll explore in this chapter. The experience and management of stress is also highly individual. As a result, it's important to pay close attention to your emotions and learn to listen to your body when it comes to stress.

Certain stressors will always be with us, but we can learn healthy ways to cope. Our goal is to help you understand stress on a biological level, and to teach you some strategies that have helped us—and others—manage stress as a part of daily life.

Stress Myths

Let's begin by addressing a few common misconceptions about stress that have been floating around for a while.

• Myth 1: Stress looks and feels the same for everyone.

The experience of stress is as varied as we are. Factors like personality type, past experiences, and environmental context can have a significant effect on our stress responses.

We all know the person who is seemingly never stressed versus the friend in constant panic mode. Stress hits people differently, and we all have different coping mechanisms. Some of us shut down or get angry in times of stress, while others become more verbal and need more external validation. It depends on the individual.

• Myth 2: Stress only occurs during major life events.

Have you ever gotten incredibly stressed over something that you know is relatively small and benign in the grand scheme of things? Maybe you spill coffee on your favorite sweater or come back to a tiny scratch on your car, and it just sets you off and ruins your entire day. We tend to expect and anticipate stress during significant life events such as moving, changing jobs, getting divorced, or dealing with serious illness.

However, stressors that arise in the form of smaller, everyday events and common irritants—traffic delays, minor work pressures, miscommunications, waiting in line—those little buggy things add up, and can have a significant impact on your overall quality of life. These small moments should not be downplayed or ignored, because we might have the most control over our response to them.

• Myth 3: Stress is always bad.

Prolonged stress, known as chronic stress, is never a great thing for your health. However, there is a type of positive stress, known as eustress, that has been shown to have health and performance benefits. When we intentionally put ourselves into manageable, short-term stress situations like a speaking engagement, an intense workout, or working under a tight deadline, we experience eustress. In these situations, the biomechanics of stress kick us into high gear, improving our alertness, energy, and concentration in short bursts. More on this on page 174.

• Myth 4: No symptoms, no stress.

While symptoms are a good indicator that stress is present, the symptoms of stress aren't always what you might expect (e.g., headache, bad sleep, low energy). Stress symptoms can manifest in many different and more subtle ways, like changes in social behavior, increased sensitivity or emotional response, and moodiness. They might not look like symptoms at all, just subtle behavioral changes.

"Until recently, I thought obsessive behaviors and other little tics were just part of my personality. It wasn't until I realized that these cycles and habits came in waves that I was able to identify them as stress and anxiety responses. I've learned a lot about stress, what it looks like and how to manage it, in the last five years."

—MEREDITH

171

TYPES OF

If we want to get a better handle on our stress, we must begin with self-awareness. Is your stress ongoing and constant? This might be a sign that you are suffering from chronic stress. Are your stress triggers associated with a specific traumatic event? If you feel that you're suffering from traumatic stress, you might want to consider therapy and some form of rehab. Is your stress cyclical, typically occurring at certain times of the month? This might mean that your stress is hormonal. Considering questions like these is important for getting a clear picture of your stress.

STRESS

Let's discuss the various types of stress.

Acute Stress

Acute stress is the type of stress we experience daily and that lasts for a limited period, activating a short-term physiological stress response. Experiences that may cause acute stress to arise include having a heated argument with your spouse, being criticized by your boss, and having a near-miss traffic accident. Acute stress activates the "fight or flight" response in our brain, but it typically does not have long-term adverse consequences. The exception is if acute stress symptoms persist for more than a month or so, which could lead to someone being diagnosed with post-traumatic stress disorder (PTSD).

Chronic Stress

This type of stress is more long-term and pervasive, typically the result of an ongoing difficult situation like extreme pressure at work, family dysfunction, or a long-term illness. This type of stress has the greatest negative impact on long-term health and can manifest in physical, emotional, and behavioral issues.

What Are the Effects?

● **Physical health:** Under chronic stress, your body releases the hormones adrenaline and cortisol, which trigger the "fight or flight" response. This response can be useful at times, but when it becomes chronic, it can lead to a wide variety of health issues. Chronic stress has also been linked to decreased immunity and hormonal imbalances.

● **Addiction issues:** Chronic stress has been linked to addiction to substances, as well as behavioral addictions, such as to the internet, food, or gambling.

● **Mental health:** Anxiety, lack of focus, fatigue, impaired memory, clouded thinking, and obsessive behavior patterns can all be signs of chronic stress. Those with chronic stress are more susceptible to developing mood and anxiety disorders.

● **Diminished quality of life:** Chronic stress makes us irritable and withdrawn, affecting our relationships at home as well as in the outside world and at work. Chronic stress is also linked to decreased productivity at work, as a stressed brain is a less clear and focused brain.

Post-traumatic Stress Disorder (PTSD)

PTSD is a psychiatric disorder that can develop in people after experiencing a traumatic event that is perceived as particularly dangerous or life threatening. Examples of traumatic experiences that can lead to PTSD include natural disasters, serious accidents, and abuse or sexual assault. It is natural to feel afraid and experience a fight or flight response during a traumatic situation. While people typically recover from acute stress over time, traumatic stress can lead to PTSD. With PTSD intense, disturbing thoughts and feelings related to the traumatic experience last long after the event is over and can range from intense flashbacks and emotional responses to persistent negative thoughts and shifts in mood.

Environmental Stress

This type of stress arises from living in unsafe conditions, including noise, pollution, extreme temperatures, crime, and war. Environmental stress can negatively impact both physical and mental health, contributing to a constant sense of discomfort or unease. Assessing stress-inducing factors in your environment is an important consideration. Although environmental stress is not always chronic, it can be.

Physiological Stress

Physiological stress refers to the body's response to internal or external stressors that disrupt homeostasis. Examples of physiological stress include illness, injury, sleep deprivation, and nutritional deficiencies, which activate physiological stress pathways in the brain and body and compromise health.

This Is Your Body on Stress

Our body's stress response is a biological survival mechanism that involves the nervous, endocrine, and immune systems all working together in unison to react to a real or perceived threat. It's called the "fight or flight" response because that's exactly what nature intended it to do—preserve our survival.

The problem in the modern world is that while most of the stress in our lives is non-life-threatening, on a neurobiological level, we experience stress the same way our hunter-gatherer ancestors did to protect them-selves from predators. Today, the repeated activation of this stress response (even in non-life-threatening situations) can lead to chronic stress.

Stress does a lot to the body that we can't necessarily see or feel immediately, and over time this can have significant long-term effects. When we perceive a threat (real or imagined), the body goes into fight or flight mode. Once the body perceives stress, the hypothalamus in the brain signals the adrenal glands to release stress hormones, primarily cortisol and adrenaline, into the bloodstream. Adrenaline increases heart rate, blood pressure, and energy—the rush you'll feel—while cortisol boosts glucose (sugar) availability in the blood, enhancing the brain's essential functions. While all this is happening, cortisol suppresses non-essential systems like digestion, immune response, and reproductive functions to conserve energy.

All these reactions make up the fight or flight response, sharpening focus and alertness. If stress is prolonged (chronic), elevated cortisol levels can lead to a long list of negative side effects. Under most acute stressful circumstances, once the perceived threat is gone, hormone levels in the body will return to normal, and the parasympa-thetic nervous system (PNS) will slow down the stress response.[2]

How Stress Affects the Body

BRAIN

- Inflammation and dysfunction that affect memory, concentration, and mood

- Increased anxiety and depression

- Brain fog

- Increased risk of headache, migraine, and stroke

CARDIOVASCULAR

- Increased blood pressure and risk of heart disease and stroke

- Higher cholesterol and triglycerides

- Atherosclerosis

DIGESTIVE SYSTEM

- Irritable bowel, bloating, pain and discomfort

- Imbalance of gut microbiota

- Bowel changes (diarrhea, constipation)

- Indigestion

IMMUNE SYSTEM

- Suppressed innate and adaptive immunity

- Altered immune cell balance and functions

- Decreased immune defenses

- Increased risk of illness

MUSCULOSKELETAL SYSTEM

- Inflammation and pain in muscles and/or joints

- Increased tension, tightness, and soreness

- Trigger points

ENDOCRINE SYSTEM

- Negative shifts in variety of hormones, including those regulating blood sugar, reproduction, fat metabolism, blood pressure, and digestion

What Is Cortisol?

Cortisol, aka the "stress hormone," is a steroid hormone produced by the adrenal glands. Cortisol is essential in regulating stress, metabolism, and immune response, and it plays a crucial role in managing these functions by helping the body respond to stress, regulate blood sugar levels, reduce inflammation, and maintain overall balance.[3]

176

Under normal conditions, cortisol production in the body follows a circadian rhythm, and cortisol levels tend to be highest for most people shortly after they wake up and lowest in the middle of the night.[4] Cortisol production increases under stress, ideally helping your body to manage through a series of responses that provide the necessary energy to cope with stressful situations.

While this response is essential at certain times, long-term elevated cortisol levels can have a cascade of adverse effects, including:

Slowing Down Metabolism: Cortisol helps manage how the body metabolizes proteins, fats, and carbohydrates. It converts these nutrients to energy, ensuring the body has enough power to function properly—especially during times of stress. If your body is under the constant influence of cortisol, it can slow down your metabolism, keeping it in preservation mode and causing weight gain.

Spiking Blood Sugar: Cortisol stimulates glucose metabolism to ensure that the body has an adequate supply of glucose needed for energy during times of stress. Chronically high levels of cortisol can lead to elevated blood sugar and can contribute to insulin resistance and type 2 diabetes.

Compromising Immune Function: Cortisol has anti-inflammatory effects and helps regulate the immune system. It can suppress inflammation and immune responses, but chronic cortisol elevation can lead to the immune system becoming "resistant." This resistance means that the immune system doesn't respond to cortisol's anti-inflammatory signals as effectively as it should. As a result, inflammation can become harder to control, leading to a heightened risk of chronic inflammatory and autoimmune diseases.[5]

Elevating Blood Pressure: Cortisol helps maintain blood pressure by balancing salt and water in the body. Chronically increased cortisol levels have been linked to hypertension.[6]

Disrupting Circadian Rhythm: Cortisol follows a twenty-four-hour cycle, rising and falling at specific times of the day. This pattern helps regulate the body's sleep-wake cycle and overall energy levels.[7] When cortisol levels are too high, the body's natural rhythms can be disrupted, leading to a wide range of negative effects. (See more in Chapter 5: Help Your Self Sleep So Good, page 146.)

Affecting Mood and Cognitive Function: Chronically high levels of cortisol are associated with depression and anxiety, and they also impact cognitive functions like memory and attention span. Elevated stress hormones may also contribute to dementia.[8]

The Rise and Fall of Cortisol

Understanding how the body's cortisol levels naturally rise and fall throughout the day is a key piece of effectively managing stress. Our cortisol naturally tends to spike between 7 and 8 a.m., right after we wake up. This peak varies among individuals and is related to when you naturally wake up—aka "the cortisol awakening response." The resulting flood of glucose creates the energy we need to get going. The flip side is that these early morning hours are also when we are most susceptible to stress. Therefore, waking up and looking at your phone or engaging in stressful discourse with your spouse (or whomever) first thing in the morning is not optimal.

Caffeine intake is another factor that can affect our morning cortisol levels. Studies show that caffeine increases cortisol secretion, which means that if you start your day with coffee first thing, your body will start to rely on the caffeine instead of producing cortisol on its own. This both interferes with our body's natural cortisol production and contributes to caffeine dependence (we then think we need the coffee to wake up). While there are benefits to moderate coffee consumption, we would recommend delaying that first cup of coffee, rather than drinking it immediately upon waking. If you allow your body the chance to wake up with its cortisol spike, drinking coffee about an hour after waking should be ideal for most people. Coffee can benefit you without disrupting your body's natural cortisol flow when consumed at the right time.

177

Is All Stress Bad?

The short answer? No, not all stress is bad.

While chronic or traumatic stress can be damaging, moderate amounts of stress can boost resilience, improve cognitive function, and be used to our benefit. **This type of positive stress, called "eustress," is defined as a type of stress that results from engaging in challenging but attainable and enjoyable tasks.** When we experience eustress, we may feel boosts of energy, creativity, focus, and motivation.

While it's convenient to separate stress into two categories—"good" (eustress) and "bad" (distress)—people can experience a stressor as both eustress and distress simultaneously. The perception of good or bad stress is highly individual and depends on many factors, including personality, past experiences, how much control one has over the situation, and environmental context. There are those of us who love nothing more than public speaking or to participate in a competitive athletic event—and there are those of us for whom these things are our worst nightmare.

Studies have shown that low and high levels of stress reactivity are linked to poorer health, whereas moderate levels of reactivity predicted better health outcomes. These findings suggest that individuals with very low or very high stress reactivity could benefit from interventions to enhance their emotional regulation and coping skills, in order to enter the "Goldilocks zone" of stress reactivity.[9]

Stress Inoculation

"I like to think of stress inoculation as a stress detox, where you increase stress to reduce stress (or improve stress response) by getting it up and out of your system. By stress inoculation, I mean forcing my body to do stressful things, like go on a long run, sit in a sauna, or take a cold plunge; you could think of it as toning yourself up to handle future stress. Either way, you'll get the idea in this section."

—MEREDITH

In modern society, our access to comfort and convenience has removed much of the acute stress that we would have encountered in the past. And yet, our mental health and emotional well-being are arguably at an all-time low. Many of us are chronically stressed. So, what can we do about it?

Our recommendation is stress inoculation, or hormesis, which is about building stress resilience: the idea that by exposing our bodies to manageable amounts of stress or discomfort, we can improve health and performance and reduce stress. Stress inoculation works a bit like a stress fitness routine, and it can help improve the body's reaction to stress on both a mental and a physical level.

Here's how it works:

ACTIVATION, ADAPTATION, AND REGULATION

By activating the stress response system with repeated, controlled exposure to stress, the body learns to regulate the HPA (hypothalamic-pituitary-adrenal) axis more efficiently. This can lead to a more balanced release of stress hormones and reduced stress intensity over time.

NEUROPLASTICITY AND MENTAL RESILIENCE

The brain undergoes structural and functional changes in response to repeated stress exposure. This exercise in neuroplasticity strengthens the neural pathways associated with stress resilience and improves the brain's ability to cope with future stressors.

IMPROVED IMMUNITY

Studies very clearly point to a positive, temporary boost in immune activity from moderate, controlled stress exposure. This controlled exposure may lead to longer-term enhanced immune function.[10]

Stress Inoculation Techniques

Here are some ways to induce stress positively. (Please note: These are tools for helping to manage stress in healthy-bodied people, so if you have any specific health concerns, please consult a physician first.)

- **PHYSICAL EXERCISE:** Strength training, HIIT training, long runs, cycling, and other high-intensity workouts.

- **EXTREME AND CONTROLLED TEMPERATURE EXPOSURE:** ice baths, cryo therapy, cold plunges, and sauna.

- **INTERMITTENT FASTING** Eating within an eight-hour window or periodic fasting.

- **MENTAL CHALLENGES** Public speaking, problem solving, and strategy games.

Exercise and Stress

Exercise is probably the most common health recommendation for physical fitness and stress reduction. While most of us recognize exercise as a form of physical fitness, we often overlook the connection between exercise, stress management, and mental health. If you're stressed, it might be hard to find time to exercise, as you put other priorities first, and this just perpetuates the cycle. If we can ask anything of you in these pages, please find the time to exercise and sweat it out, even if it's once a week.

Here's how exercise works to moderate your stress levels:

The intensity of exercise influences the body's stress response system, specifically the HPA axis, in a way that is dependent on the level of exertion. Higher-intensity exercise = greater release of cortisol. This increased cortisol release from intense exercise can, in turn, reduce the amount of cortisol that is released in response to later psychological stress. In other words, you handle stress better. Exercising intensely can make the body less reactive to future stress by initially elevating cortisol levels and dampening the response to subsequent stressors.[11] The harder you work out, the more cortisol is released and the less it shows up in unwanted scenarios.

If you menstruate, try to manage your workouts according to your menstrual cycle. For many women, energy levels are highest during the follicular phase—the phase between your period and ovulation. Maximizing on that energy spike can feel good and set you up for success later in your cycle when you might feel less energetic.

Mindfulness and Stress

Practicing mindfulness is both the most challenging and the easiest way to cope with stress. In a fast-paced, forward-thinking world, it is tough to slow down and stay focused on the present moment. When we say mindfulness, we are speaking about breaking the cycle of stress that often stems from worrying about the future or dwelling on the past. An attempt to stay fully present. This practice allows us to understand our stress triggers and responses better and creates space for more thoughtful reactions. We can practice mindfulness by engaging in any activity that allows us to slow down and stay present, from meditation to taking a calming walk in nature. And what's the one thing we shouldn't do when it comes to a mindfulness practice? Overthink it.

Meditation

Meditation is often the hardest stress-management technique to make time for. Many of us are addicted to momentum and have a tough time sitting still. Meditation emphasizes the importance of stillness and focus, which are the opposite of how most of us spend our time. However, it is an important and highly effective way of managing stress, and we recommend finding time for it, even if it's just ten minutes a day. Meditation is defined as the focusing of the mind to achieve a state of mental clarity, emotional calmness, and heightened awareness, and can involve various techniques such as deep breathing, guided imagery, or mantra repetition, all of which help quiet the mind and bring us to a state of attention.

A substantial amount of research links meditation practices to improved mental health and well-being by reducing the biomarkers typically associated with stress—cortisol, heart rate variability (HRV), blood pressure, and inflammatory cytokines. Studies also suggest that meditation alleviates distress from psychological stressors by influencing key psychological processes, reducing activation in brain regions involved in rumination (overthinking, obsessing) and improving mood regulation.

Time Spent in Nature

The easiest form of meditation for us is finding time to spend in nature. When you are able to take a long walk outside, hike, have a beach day, or just simply find a quiet spot in the grass, this can do wonders for your nervous system. Time spent outside can be a form of meditation, as it naturally encourages mindfulness and presence in the moment. The sensory experiences—the feel of the breeze, the sight of a natural landscape, the sound of water—all draw our attention away from daily distractions, and help quiet the mind, much like traditional meditation practices.

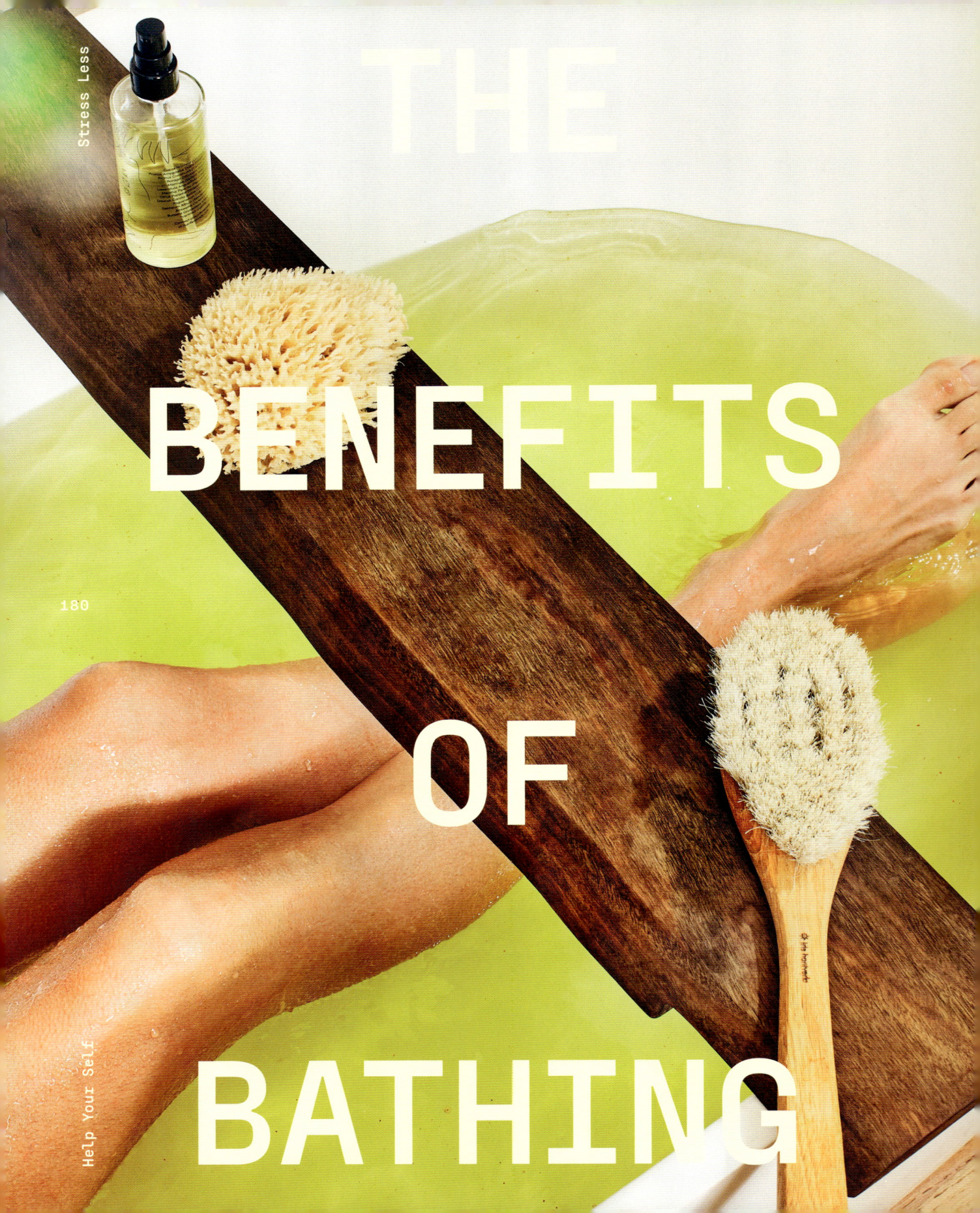

THE

BENEFITS

OF

BATHING

"

It's almost a joke around our house how much I love to bathe. At some point in my mid-life, I realized that starting the day with a relaxing bath could feel as good or effective as exercise as a stress management tool. Sometimes the baths I take are truly relaxing, with essential oils, a good book, and the whole ambient thing. Other times, what feels most relaxing is dictating a few emails and checking a few things off the to-do list instead of letting it build up and swim around in my head. While I recognize the latter might not sound super relaxing, it works for me.

—MEREDITH

Many of us are addicted to constant movement. During a typical busy day, who has time for a bath? The health benefits might convince you otherwise. Bathing is not just about personal preference. Studies have shown that bathing benefits us by raising our internal body temperature, leading to enhanced circulation, which delivers oxygen and nutrients to the body's extremities and helps remove metabolic waste.

In a study that compared the health effects of immersion bathing versus showering, results showed that bathing significantly improved stress, pain, and fatigue scores and increased overall well-being compared with showering. Participants also reported better general and mental health, emotional role functioning, and social functioning.[12]

I didn't need an excuse to bathe more—what about you?

181

Ingestibles for Stress

"

I'll be the first to admit that I didn't believe much in the science of ingestibles to reduce stress. Even with all my knowledge and research, I still associated stress with specific situations and considered it less about my reactions. So, for me, stress reduction "looked" a certain way, like a glass of wine, a nice meal, a massage, a workout, a day at the beach—you name it. While all these things can be temporarily relaxing, it wasn't until recently that I started to "feel" what supplements could do for my stress levels. Fortunately, there is so much amazing science behind them.

—MEREDITH

I was always hesitant to take adaptogens because of concerns about their safety, as well as their potency. More emerging science also needed to be developed. That has changed a lot in the last few years. Many higher-quality ingredients are safer to take, and more studies are coming out every day. It's made me more confident to explore ingredients that can profoundly impact my mood.

—KAT

Ashwagandha

If you've been into wellness at all, you've probably come across ashwagandha by now. It's an adaptogenic herb that's been a staple in Ayurvedic and indigenous medicine for more than three thousand years. Also known as "Indian Ginseng" or "Winter Cherry," this small shrub comes from regions in India, Pakistan, and parts of Africa. It's part of the same plant family as potatoes and tomatoes. The name "ashwagandha" means "horse's smell" in Sanskrit, which comes from the scent of its fresh root. The herb is famous for its ability to help the body manage stress and keep things balanced, particularly by regulating cortisol levels.

Ashwagandha acts as an adaptogen, meaning it helps the body adapt to stress and maintain balance. It helps regulate cortisol levels by influencing the body's stress response system, particularly the hypothalamic-pituitary-adrenal (HPA) axis, which is responsible for managing how the body reacts to stress. Over time this helps prevent the negative effects of chronic stress and promotes a more balanced and resilient stress response.[13]

Saffron

Relatively new to the supplement scene, saffron is a spice derived from the *Crocus sativus L.* plant, which belongs to the botanical family that includes the species Iris, Freesia, and Gladiolus.

Although saffron has been used for more than four thousand years in foods, beverages, dyes, dietary supplements, and cosmetics, it has most recently been used primarily as a gourmet spice. Its unique flavor is hard to define when compared to other spices—lightly sweet but earthy—and it is versatile enough to be used in both sweet and savory applications.

As a spice, it is great, but as a supplement, it is potentially revolutionary.

Studies have shown that saffron extract appears to reduce depressive mood in healthy individuals, contributing to the large body of evidence supporting the benefits of saffron on depression outcomes in both clinical and nonclinical populations. Notably, this study is the first to demonstrate the beneficial effect of saffron on heart rate variability in response to a psychosocial stressor, indicating that saffron may enhance resilience against the development of stress-related psychiatric disorders. Further research is needed to elucidate the exact mechanisms underlying these effects.[14]

L-theanine

L-theanine is an amino acid primarily found in tea (Camellia sinensis) and a few other plants, such as the edible mushroom Imleria badia. Tea is considered the primary dietary source of L-theanine. Keep in mind that we're speaking about tea leaves—black, green, white, oolong, etc.—not herbal tisanes. The L-theanine content of a cup of tea varies based on the type of tea leaves, the processing, and preparation method.[15]

Although all teas contain L-theanine, based on these studies, a person would need to drink about 25 cups of green tea or about 8 cups of black tea per day to get 200 mg of L-theanine, widely considered the therapeutic dose.[16] This is why we prefer to take it in supplemental form, along with regular tea consumption.

Due to its well-studied calming and stress-relieving properties, L-theanine has the potential to be developed into an effective nutraceutical. Specifically, it could help alleviate and prevent mental confusion and stress-related issues, making it a valuable ingredient in promoting mental well-being.[17]

The antistress effects of L-theanine at 200 mg per day have been demonstrated with both once-daily and twice-daily administration. Its benefits for improving attention have been observed with a daily intake of 100 mg over four days and a single 200 mg dose, supported by decreased responses in functional magnetic resonance imaging (fMRI).[18] Additionally, L-theanine has shown potential therapeutic effects in psychiatric disorders. Studies have also reported multiple positive effects of a four-week regimen of L-theanine (250 mg/day) in patients with major depressive disorder (MDD). However, this was based on an open-label study.

THE ROUTINE

Going deeper into a stress reduction routine requires combining the techniques we've discussed in this chapter in a way that works for you. We can't emphasize enough the importance of doing what feels right for you and your lifestyle. Below are some of the daily habits that work for us, and what we have found to be consistently effective.

● **6:00**AM (PUT YOUR PHONE IN AIRPLANE MODE)

When you wake up, your cortisol is at its highest. Putting your phone on airplane mode is a game changer for not waking up to a slew of messages and alerts that may have come in overnight. It can all wait until you're ready.

184

● **7:00**AM (ADAPTOGENS IN THE MORNING)

We love a good mix of L-theanine, saffron, and ashwagandha in supplement form. This combo is a life-changing way to start the day.

● **8:00**AM (ALTERNATING-INTENSITY WORKOUT)

We've already established that physical activity is one of the most effective ways to manage stress and boost mood, and it is the go-to for both of us to keep sane.

● **12:00**PM (STAY CONNECTED)

For many of us, our first impulse when we are stressed is to retreat. While solo time is an essential part of stress management, connecting with others is equally important, and an essential aspect of feeling good. Friends and loved ones are often the best therapists! If you work from home, try mixing it up and going to a cafe for lunch or a work session. And be sure to occasionally take meetings, especially if they have a social aspect.

On a biological level, positive social interactions with friends or loved ones trigger the release of oxytocin, often referred to as the "love hormone." Oxytocin has been shown to reduce stress and anxiety by counteracting the effects of cortisol, even if it's a quick fifteen-minute call to a friend across the country.

● **2:00**PM (SHIFT TO GRATITUDE)

We often focus so much on what isn't working during the day that we rarely lean into what is. There is a science to gratitude, and we love writing a few notes down during the day, sending a text to someone we love, or taking a brief moment to focus on what brings us joy and gratitude.

● **6:00**PM (CHANGE OF WARDROBE)

Something happens when you remove your "work" clothes and change into something cozy for the home. There may be no science here, but it is an excellent way to shift modes mentally.

● **7:00**PM (MAGNESIUM AND TART CHERRY COCKTAIL)

Instead of an alcoholic beverage, we like to wind down with something that relaxes muscles and tells our body it's time to stop eating, it's time for rest and relaxation.

● **9:00**PM (WASH THE DAY OFF)

We believe that bathing or showering at the end of the day is essential to a good night's sleep.

● **10:00**PM (DEEP SLEEP)

Getting enough sleep and having a regular sleep schedule is crucial in managing stress. Quality rest is an important aspect of feeling energized and less overwhelmed, and it also helps regulate hormones and energy cycles. We discuss how to get the best sleep in Chapter 5: Help Your Self Sleep So Good (page 146).

The conditions of modern life fight against our body's ability to regulate stress—from constant stimulation in the online world to working in offices isolated from nature—and they aren't going anywhere anytime soon.

However, we hope that through this chapter you have begun to understand that stress is not just circumstantial, caused by external factors. It is chemical, hormonal, and behavioral—and it's about what's going on inside.

Even in modern life, we do have power over how we respond to stress and live with a greater sense of calm and ease. And what we choose to put into our bodies can have a big impact on the stress we experience. Foods that help with stress are typically nutrient-dense and well balanced, and provide the body with essential vitamins and minerals to support a calm mind and stable energy levels.

Enjoy!

The Recipes

186

→ Avocado Cocoa Mousse

→ Pumpkin Seed Buckwheat Granola

Avocado Cocoa Mousse with Cinnamon

"Avocado chocolate mousse is one of the best kept secrets in the raw food repertoire. If you've never tried it, you'll probably end up wondering where it's been all your life—and yes, kids love it. I've perfected my version over the years with just the right amount of everything."

—MEREDITH

SERVES 4

2 ripe medium avocados, peeled and pitted (a perfect use for overripe avocados)

½ cup (50 g) unsweetened cocoa powder

½ cup (120 ml) maple syrup

⅓ cup (75 ml) almond milk or any plant-based milk

1 teaspoon ground cinnamon

1 teaspoon pure vanilla extract

Pinch sea salt, plus more to taste, if needed

Cacao nibs or cacao powder, for garnish

How to make?

In a blender, process the avocado, cocoa powder, maple syrup, milk, cinnamon, vanilla, and sea salt together until smooth.

Adjust for salt and sweetener if desired.

Serve the mousse in parfait glasses or small bowls. Garnish with cacao nibs or cacao powder.

Store in an airtight container in the refrigerator for up to 3 days.

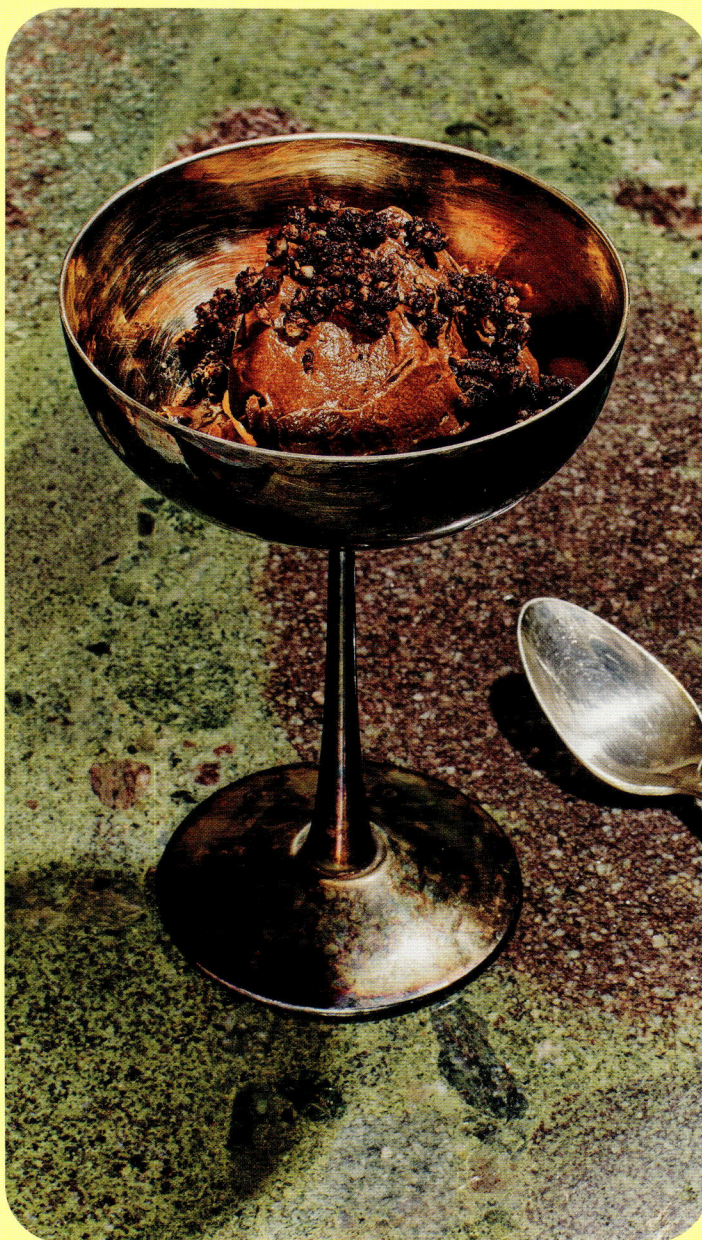

Salty-Sweet Pumpkin Seed Buckwheat Granola

Granola has always been my go-to for a snack. Most granolas on the market are made with questionable oils and too much sugar. Fortunately, making your own is actually really easy, and it keeps well.

This granola recipe is a stress buster, not only because it's rich in fiber and protein to keep you satiated, but also because it has that crispy crunch to curb any stress-induced cravings.

We recommend doubling this recipe, as it keeps for up to two months in an airtight container at room temperature.

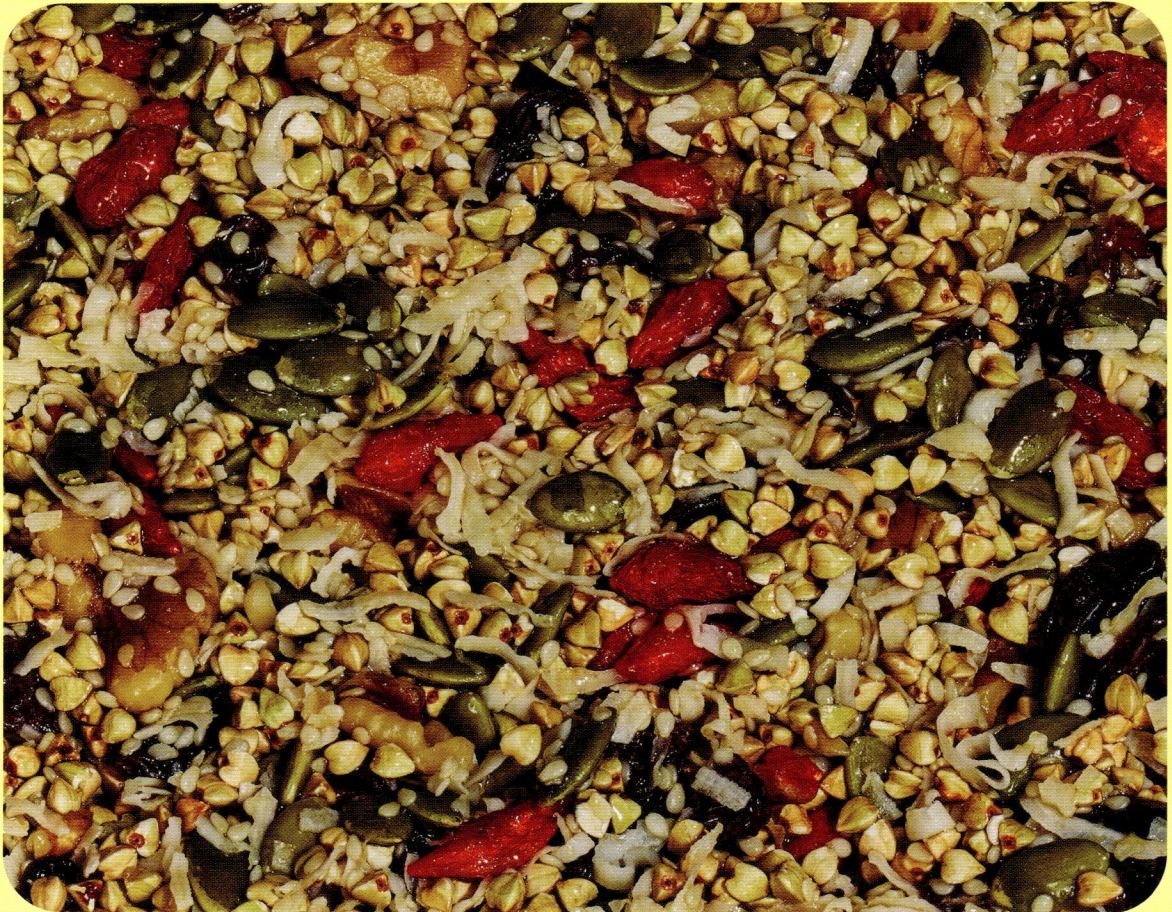

MAKES ABOUT
5 CUPS (650 G)

———————————

2 cups (350 g) buckwheat groats, soaked in water to cover overnight (not kasha)

1 cup (90 g) gluten-free old-fashioned rolled oats

1 cup (130 g) raw hulled pumpkin seeds

½ cup (75 g) sesame seeds

½ cup (60 g) walnuts, chopped

½ cup (45 g) unsweetened shredded coconut

⅓ cup (120 ml) maple syrup or honey

¼ cup (60 ml) avocado oil, olive oil, or melted coconut oil

1 teaspoon pure vanilla extract

1 teaspoon ground cinnamon or more to taste

1 teaspoon ground nutmeg or more to taste

1 teaspoon ground ginger or more to taste

1½ teaspoons ground sea salt or more to taste

½ cup (75 g) raisins or dried fruit of your choice (chop if pieces are large)

How to make?

Preheat the oven to 325°F (165°C). If your oven runs hot, set it to 300°F (150°C). Line a baking sheet with parchment paper.

In a large bowl, combine the buckwheat, oats, pumpkin seeds, sesame seeds, walnuts, and shredded coconut.

In a bowl or liquid measuring cup, whisk together the maple syrup, oil, vanilla extract, cinnamon, nutmeg, ginger, and sea salt.

Pour the wet ingredients into the dry ingredients and mix to thoroughly combine. Taste and add a little more salt or spices if you'd like.

Using a spatula, spread out the granola mixture evenly on the lined baking sheet. Bake for 25 to 30 minutes, stirring halfway through to ensure even baking.

Remove from the oven when the granola is golden brown. (The hardest part about making granola at home is making sure you don't burn it. Keep a close eye on it during the last 5 to 10 minutes of baking to ensure it does not burn.)

Allow the granola to cool on the baking sheet because it will continue to crisp up.

Once cooled, stir in the raisins. Serve over yogurt, with your favorite milk and fruit, or our favorite way—eating it on its own!

Store in an airtight container for up to 2 months for optimal freshness.

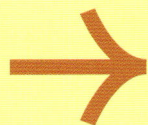

Have Better Sex

" I went to a women's entrepreneurial event when I was pregnant, and one of the keynote speakers said that her morning routine, after dropping her kids off to school, was listening to sexy audio books and getting a little spiced up on the way home. By the time she got home she was usually in the mood to have a tryst with her husband, then get to work. This was so refreshing and out of the box for the event, I just fell in love with the idea.

Sexual health isn't just about having sex—I believe it's about lighting yourself up in ways that turn you on, both literally and figuratively.
—MEREDITH

As working moms in our forties, sex can often take a backseat on the priority list for a variety of reasons, many of them having to do with time management and energy levels, not necessarily lack of desire. But sexual health is a fundamental part of overall health and accessing that energy and vitality can bring about many aspects of positive change in your life.

Reigniting sexual desire or improving your sexual health can lead to a range of positive changes, including improved mood and emotional well-being, thanks to the release of endorphins and oxytocin during sexual activity.

Sex can also enhance intimacy and connection in relationships. Physically, increased sexual activity can boost cardiovascular health, improve sleep, and even strengthen the immune system.

While we've been taught by the media that sexual expression is a sign of freedom and liberation and is something that's easy to tap into, most would agree that it's a little more complicated than that. Whether you are single or in an intimate relationship, feeling good in your body, mind, and spirit are all essential ingredients to a healthy sex life. Its significance extends beyond sexual activity, reflecting various aspects of physical, mental, and emotional health.

While other chapters in this book apply equally to all genders, this chapter is based on our experience and identity as women. While this advice is applicable to anyone, and good overall health leads to good sexual health, we want to make the distinction, as we can only write from our personal experiences. We also want to state upfront that the very basis of a healthy sex life starts with safe and consensual sex. These parameters should be a given.

We've included this chapter last because in many ways, a healthy sex life can only be established if all the other factors in this book are addressed.

With that said, lighting up your desire can light up so many other aspects of your life.

Let's Talk About Libido

"For most women, sex drive has more to do with what's going on in the brain than anything else; lower dopamine and higher serotonin levels, too many things on the mind and the plate can make getting in the mood harder. In my experience, finding ways to get out of your head and into your body drastically improves libido."

—MEREDITH

"Libido" is the psychological term for our sex drive. When we talk about libido, it tends to be with a bit of a smirk, or else in simplistic terms, leaving out the biological, mental, and emotional factors that influence sexual desire. But the truth is that libido is a complex, nuanced thing, and it is widely variable from one person to the next. For some of us, sex once a month is plenty, while for others, we want it at least once a week. It is also healthy and normal for our sex drive to shift and change throughout the stages of life.

Like many other aspects of health, libido is not a one-size-fits-all equation, with one clear definition. Its inner workings involve a complex and intricate network of hormones, environmental stimuli, emotional responses, and pleasure and reward feedback loops. It's time for a quick biology lesson on how the brain functions to regulate our sex drive.

Hormone Regulation

The brain's hypothalamus is at the center of libido regulation, responding to hormonal and neural signals and interacting with neurotransmitters like dopamine to influence sexual motivation and arousal. Sex hormones like testosterone and estrogen are regulated by other hormones secreted in the hypothalamus, primarily through the secretion of gonadotropin-releasing hormone (GnRH). GnRH stimulates the pituitary gland to release luteinizing hormone (LH) and follicle-stimulating hormone (FSH), which all work together to regulate the production of the sex hormones, testosterone and estrogen. Both testosterone and estrogen regulate libido, with testosterone being most closely linked to sex drive.[1]

The pleasure and reward feedback loop is an essential part of libido and sexual arousal, with dopamine (the "feel good" hormone) being the key player. Studies have shown that increased dopamine activity in specific brain regions directly corresponds to increased libido response.

The hypothalamus also produces and releases oxytocin (the "love hormone") and vasopressin, which are involved in sexual behavior, bonding, and emotional responses related to sexual activity. Dopamine—the source of pleasure, reward, and motivation—is involved in this process as well, and plays a key role in sexual satisfaction, overall relationship dynamics, and forming partner preferences.[2]

Processing Sensory Information

Despite its fundamental role in human life and procreation, little research has gone into the way our brains control our sexual behavior. We know that the hypothalamus processes sensory information related to sexual stimuli in the form of what we see, touch, taste, and smell. Still, we don't understand much about how responses to this vary from one person to the next.

We also know that there are differences between the way that men versus women respond to sexual stimuli. Research has revealed that when shown erotic visual stimuli, men generally experience significantly higher activation in the thalamus and hypothalamus—and hence greater sexual arousal—than women.[3] This is probably in part where the myth that men have higher sex drives than women comes from.

Autonomic Nervous System

The hypothalamus regulates the autonomic nervous system, which controls physiological responses during sexual activity, such as increased heart rate, blood flow to genital areas, and muscle contractions. In both men and women, these autonomic effects include the vascular dilation that leads to penile or clitoral erection, stimulation of secretions, and contractions of the pelvic muscles accompanying orgasm.[4]

MYTHS AND TRUTHS

The libido is complex, and sex drive can vary widely from one person to the next. This may be why there are so many myths and misunderstandings surrounding the libido. We'd like to help dispel some of them.

SURROUNDING

LIBIDO

● *Myth: Libido Declines with Age*

This is not inherently true. While hormonal shifts that happen with age can decrease libido, many people experience an increase in sexual desire as they age. This myth is most often assigned to women, and the notion that women's sex drive universally drops off in midlife while men's remains steady is oversimplified. For women, libido can fluctuate significantly due to hormonal changes during perimenopause and menopause, with some women experiencing a decrease in desire, while others may see little change or even an increase. Men do typically experience a more gradual decline in testosterone, which can affect libido over time and may be less noticeable at first, but this varies widely among individuals.

It is not accurate to say that one gender universally experiences a sharp decline while the other doesn't. Physical health and psychological well-being play the most significant role in libido throughout life for both men and women.

● *Myth: Low Libido Equals Relationship Problems*

With good communication, compassion, and understanding, a healthy relationship should be able to withstand shifts in libido. If it can't, we should be looking into other areas of the relationship. Lowered libido is not inherently an indicator of a relationship problem and is often more indicative of other lifestyle factors that prevent arousal. With that said, it is important to communicate with your partner when it comes to sexual drive and desire. Communication with mutual compassion and understanding is the key to withstanding the very natural ebbs and flows of libido throughout a long-term relationship.

● *Myth: Libido Is Strictly Hormonally Driven*

Hormones are just one small contributing factor to our libido. Just as significant are stress, mood, mental health, and environmental factors like clutter and lack of privacy.

● *Myth: Only Men Experience High Libido*

Sexual desire is an individual experience, and while some aspects of it can be correlated to gender, high libido isn't one of them. Although testosterone is closely linked to libido, its correlation to sex drive is still highly individual.

● *Myth: Libido Should Always Be High*

On the contrary, a healthy libido is dynamic, variable, and fluctuates throughout life.

● *Truth: Libido Can Be Influenced by Health Conditions*

Our overall health influences our libido, and while a lower libido does not necessarily indicate a health issue, it is crucial to assess what feels normal and healthy for you. Many medical conditions and the medications used to treat them can negatively impact libido. Discussing these side effects with a medical professional is essential if you feel this may be the case.

● *Truth: Psychological Factors Play a Significant Role in Libido*

For many people, the psychological factors involved in libido and arousal are big issues. Stress, anxiety, depression, and relationship problems can all impact libido. Modern living works against most couples in this regard.

● *Truth: Libido Varies Across Individuals*

We've established that sexual desire is highly individualized. What is normal or satisfying for one person may differ for another. Understanding and respecting differences in libido within relationships is vital for maintaining intimacy and communication.

● *Truth: Communication Is Key*

Open and honest communication about sexual needs, desires, and expectations is essential for maintaining a satisfying sexual relationship. More open communication can be a huge step toward increasing intimacy and libido.

● *Truth: Libido Can Change Over Time*

Libido fluctuates, and paying attention can inform you about your mental, physical, and emotional health. Recognizing and adapting to these changes can help individuals and couples navigate their journey.

Good Sex at Any Age

Here is our call to release the taboos! While the media does a fantastic job of misrepresenting what sex looks like—two attractive people having the most satisfying sex of their lives on the first night—you've probably figured out this isn't the case.

In real life, sex is about navigating phases and tuning in to our bodies—things may feel sexier at some times than at others. The goal of this section is to help you understand that there are both physiological and psychological factors at play, and these factors are directly impacted by our current phases of life.

TUNING IN

No matter what phase of life you are in, having sex can be a time to connect. Sex can be a profound opportunity to engage with ourselves and our partner(s) on a deeper, more conscious level. Unlike the many routine moments in our daily lives, sex is inherently intimate, urging us to be fully present physically and emotionally. This experience, when approached mindfully, can open up a space to listen and feel.

Tuning in during sex allows us to connect with our own needs and desires, recognize areas of tension or vulnerability, and foster a sense of safety and openness with our partner. The act of slowing down and paying attention to sensations, breathing, and shared energy can deepen intimacy, amplify trust, and cultivate a stronger connection—not just with another person but also with ourselves. In this way, sex becomes more than a physical act; it's a practice in mindfulness and self-awareness, creating space for growth, healing, and connection.

SEX AND PREGNANCY

Trying to get pregnant can involve having lots of sex and sharing intimacy. If you are new to the adventure, try to not let ovulation windows and calendar dates get in the way. The more sex the better during this phase, to increase the chance of getting pregnant. But when pregnancy is the goal, timelines and impatience can take over enjoying sex. Many people find the experience of trying to get pregnant to be very unsexy, especially if fertility issues are involved. If this is you, it is time to be gentle with yourself, as stress doesn't help with fertility. Try to keep it as light as possible. This is a time when communication and trust are vital.

POSTPARTUM

This phase is twofold. For one, there is so much mainstream communication that tells you that your sex drive will go off a cliff postpartum, that you won't be attracted to your partner, and all you'll think about is your baby. Postpartum sex can be complicated—tiny baby possibly in your bed, exhaustion, nursing, hormonal shifts, etc. But the death of your sex drive doesn't have to be a given. Seeing a baby brought to life with someone you love can also feel satisfying and increase your physical and emotional bond. Lean into that if you can!

If you are postpartum, and finding yourself completely devoid of a sex drive, understand that this is also very normal—and it will most likely return once you get more sleep.

PARENTING

Once you get past the postpartum phase and are parenting young children, your sex life can enter what looks like a "maintenance" phase. School, work, schedules, weekend activities, birthdays—the list of duties for young parents goes on and on. This is when it becomes vital to work sex into your schedule and make time to connect. Date nights, weekly check-ins, workouts together, and hanging out without your children can be great ways to establish connection, communication, and intimacy with your partner. You may find that one partner wants to have sex to connect, and the other needs to communicate and connect to get in the mood. Making space for both approaches is essential.

PERIMENOPAUSE

This word is having a moment. Five years ago, no one was talking about perimenopause, but it seems that now everyone is. Perimenopause is defined as the phase when a woman's body undergoes hormonal changes, particularly a decline in estrogen and progesterone levels. It can last several years and may involve irregular periods, hot flashes, mood swings, and changes in sleep patterns. It typically occurs when a woman is in her forties, but it can start earlier or later.

There is, of course, no one way to describe sex during this phase of a woman's life. For some women, their drive may spike, and for others, it may drastically decline, and she may experience vaginal dryness, discomfort during sex, and decreased libido. We believe that managing the other aspects of our health—particularly stress—is essential to successfully navigating this phase without too many drastic life changes.

MENOPAUSE

At the end of perimenopause, menopause is the culmination of all these hormonal changes that women go through. Menopause is defined as the time in a woman's life when she permanently stops menstruating, marking the end of her reproductive years. It is officially diagnosed after a woman has gone twelve consecutive months without a menstrual period. The psychological and emotional aspects of this phase can be challenging to navigate, but many women also go through it seamlessly.

When it comes to navigating sex during menopause, the steep decline in estrogen can cause symptoms that include vaginal dryness, decreased libido, issues with arousal, and an overall decrease in desire, but this does not have to be the case. Many women have pleasant experiences with menopause and enjoy not having a period! Don't psych yourself out with fear; take action by taking good care of yourself.

In many ways, all the chapters in this book can positively influence your sex drive, especially during menopause. By regulating stress, improving digestion, and sleep, we can regulate the hormonal changes that happen during this phase and the transition can be less intense.

Open communication with your partner is key, and discussing what feels good or what might need adjustment can relieve any pressure and build intimacy. Exploring different types of lubrication, new positions, or focusing more on foreplay can enhance comfort and pleasure. Practicing mindfulness can also make each touch and sensation more meaningful, helping you stay present and fully engaged. Embracing this time as a chance to rediscover your body and prioritize self-care can lead to fulfilling, satisfying sexual experiences that honor where you are in life.

Throughout all these life transitions, we cannot stress enough how important it is to focus on emotional intimacy and communication. Your overall health and well-being will determine how smooth these transitions are.

How Much Sex Is Normal?

One of the biggest questions that many of us have regarding sexual health is how much sex is normal, especially in long-term relationships. Our answer: The optimal amount of sex is whatever you define as optimal within your relationship.

With that said, research has shown that frequent, healthy sexual activity, which often includes orgasms, can have positive effects on overall physical and mental health. Physically, orgasms release endorphins and oxytocin, which help reduce stress, enhance mood, and promote relaxation. Some studies have indicated that having sex at least once a week for most couples improves and increases relationship quality and satisfaction. So, the health benefits are there, and the importance of healthy intimacy for physical, mental, and emotional health cannot be overlooked—but there is no specific number.

It is also interesting to note that, in general, studies have shown that people are having less sex than they did in past decades. This may come as a surprise or even sound like a good thing if you are a parent and worried about what your preteens or teenagers are doing with their friends. However, we believe this decline is another example of natural and healthy behaviors being disrupted by the demands of modern life. Several factors contribute to this trend, including increased work stress, longer working hours, the pervasive use of technology (smartphones and social media), and changing social dynamics. Additionally, a decline in general relationship satisfaction and intimacy can also be factored in. However, the impact varies widely based on individual circumstances.[5]

Vaginal Health

We can't speak about sexual health without addressing vaginal well-being. While vaginal health is typically a reflection of our overall health, there are some specific things we can do to care for our lady parts and to better understand what is going on down there. Proper hygiene, staying hydrated, using gentle, nonirritating products, and wearing the appropriate undergarments can all help to support our sexual health by preventing infections and discomfort. Vaginal health is like gut health in many vital ways, with good bacteria being critical to a healthy environment. If you are taking care of your digestive health, most of the time, your vaginal health will also be in order.

198

Here are some of the most important considerations when caring for your vagina.

Microbial balance

Vaginal well-being relies on maintaining an ideal balance of beneficial bacteria in the vagina. Lactobacillus species are predominant in the vagina, producing lactic acid to maintain an acidic pH, which protects against infections.

An imbalance in the body's overall microbiome, known as dysbiosis, can lead to health issues in both the gut and the vagina. Dysbiosis is typically caused by factors including sexual activity, hormonal changes, stress, overuse of antibiotics, and occasionally, hygiene practices. In the gut, dysbiosis can cause digestive problems, while in the vagina, it can lead to infections like bacterial vaginosis or yeast infections.

Probiotic use

Our vaginal microbiomes vary based on cultural, behavioral, and genetic factors. Taking probiotics can help maintain or restore a healthy balance of bacteria in both the gut and vagina.

The most prominent and beneficial strain of bacteria in the vaginal microbiome are strains of lactobacilli. Lactobacillus is the predominant microorganism in the vagina and plays a crucial role by preserving the mucosal barrier and preventing infections. To support a healthy balance of these beneficial bacteria, you can consume probiotic-rich foods or take supplements. Foods like yogurt, kefir, sauerkraut, kimchi, and other fermented products are excellent natural sources of probiotics, including Lactobacillus strains. While supplements can also be effective, getting probiotics through food may provide additional nutrients and a broader range of beneficial bacteria.[6] We would recommend getting a diverse array of probiotics from both supplements and food sources, especially if you suffer from frequent yeast infections or UTIs.

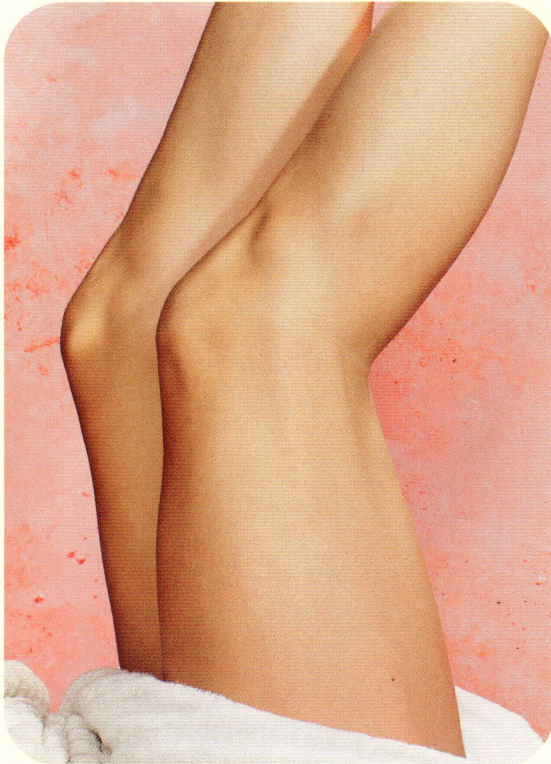

Immune health

Vaginal health and immune health are closely interconnected, as a healthy immune system helps maintain the balance of the vaginal microbiome, preventing infections and inflammation. When the immune system is compromised, this balance can be disrupted, making the body more susceptible to bacterial infection, yeast infections, and sexually transmitted diseases.

Diet and lifestyle practices

Like the gut, a balanced diet rich in fiber, probiotics, and prebiotics supports vaginal health and a healthy vaginal microbiome. We know that there are a variety of devices, sprays, creams, and supplements out there marketed for vaginal health. We generally stand by the philosophy that less is best regarding these products. If you aren't experiencing any issues, it is best to wash with a gentle cleanser and leave things alone down there. If you are experiencing a problem of any sort, consult with your gynecologist before you do anything.

Proper clothing

When it comes to maintaining vaginal health and avoiding issues like yeast infections, we recommend choosing natural fibers and properly fitting garments (nothing too tight), and focusing on what makes you most comfortable. Tight synthetic underwear isn't going to do anyone any favors.

Sex toys and tools

Sex toys have exited the area of taboo and have gone entirely mainstream—now being represented in all manner of shapes, colors, sizes, and packaging that is targeted toward women who aren't necessarily heading to the sex shops in their spare time. While we appreciate the trend and see them as valuable tools to spice things up when needed or as a healthy way of sexual exploration, we feel that overreliance on them can reduce the authentic intimacy that comes from partnered intercourse. Of course, these tools can be used in tandem, and if that pleases you, we're all for it.

Waxing and hair removal

No-hair-down-there (or almost none) has been on trend for a long time. We don't need to get into the stylistic reasons or preferences as we really don't have an opinion, but the truth is, women have hair down there for a reason. Being overly focused on waxing and hair removal can negatively impact your sex life in several ways, including skin irritation, pain and discomfort, increased sensitivity (the bad kind), and decreased sensitivity (the good kind). While we understand maintenance, we'd recommend being gentle with this area and not overly focused on it in the looks department. Being insecure about the hair on your vagina is not going to improve your sex life because—big secret—no one cares; nor should they.

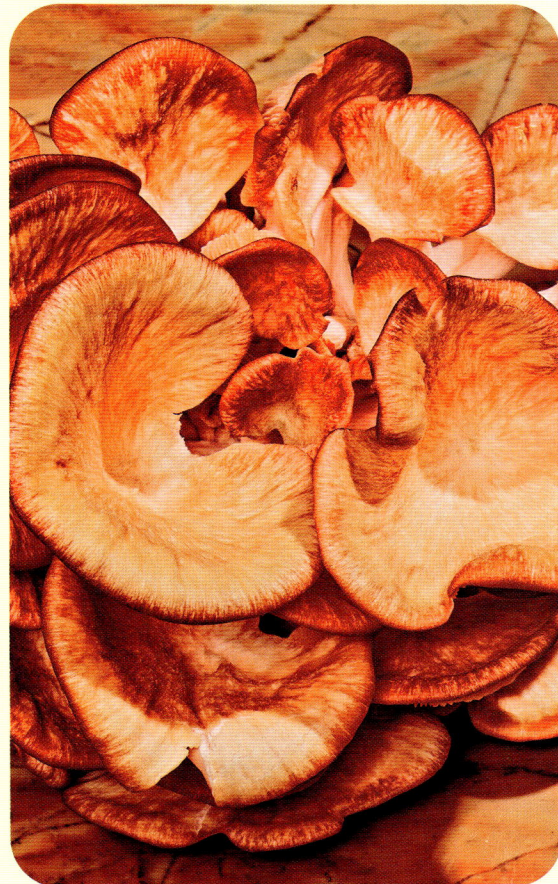

199

Relationship Building

"

Communication is the key to boosting intimacy in ways that most of us don't realize. This doesn't necessarily mean talking about sex, which, honestly, often feels to me like an intimacy killer. Instead, what I've found through personal experience is that the kind of communication that leads to good sex is about connecting and getting to know one another again. Especially for couples with small children or those who have been together for a long time, so much of our communication becomes logistical, and we stop generating conversation that inspires intimacy. I've found that it is vital in my marriage to continue seeing, respecting, and being intimate with one another.

—MEREDITH

One of our favorite quotes about the importance of communication to intimacy is from psychotherapist Sharon Loeschen:

"Communication is to relationships what breath is to life."

We could not agree more, and in this section, we want to move away from the physical aspects of sexual health into the emotional. Sex, as we know, is so much more than a physical act, and in fact, the relational side of sexual health is just as important as the physical.

Deep, physical, and satisfying connections come with relationship building, which is an ongoing process, especially in long-term relationships. Extensive literature exists on the impact of relationship satisfaction on overall well-being, showing that fulfilling romantic relationships contribute to happiness and health. In contrast, unsatisfying ones can harm mental health and even affect mortality.[7] Building healthy relationships is one of the most important things we'll discuss in this book and can influence every other factor of our well-being.

Backed by neuroscience and supported by personal experience, these are some of the most helpful ways to enhance communication in intimate relationships:

COMMUNICATION DEEPENS CONNECTION

The start of a relationship may feel natural or effortless for many of us, driven by passion and physical attraction. However, that new relationship energy eventually fades, meaning maintaining a long-term connection with a partner requires concentrated effort and enhanced communication skills. Better communication leads to more profound emotional connection, which in turn builds both emotional and physical intimacy, leading to sex that can feel more fulfilling and meaningful. Practice those communication skills so you and your partner feel safe, heard, seen, and supported.

If we had all the answers that made communication between couples easy, we would have solved one of the biggest problems between partners. We can only offer a few simple tools that have worked for us in our marriages.

ACTIVE LISTENING

This is a big one. When we've spent a long time in a relationship, it's easy to jump to conclusions or tune the other person out. Staying fully engaged when your partner is trying to communicate with you is essential in maintaining the emotional bond. Listen. And listen with empathy.

REGULAR CHECK-INS OR USING COMMUNICATION CARDS

We are big fans of using prompt cards designed explicitly for relationship communication. These are simple card decks with questions on them to open up talking points. So much communication becomes transactional, especially in long-term relationships, and these cards can help shift the narrative. It may sound cheesy at first, but once you open up and talk about things when prompted, it feels liberating and works wonders in reestablishing communication skills. A regular night can almost start to feel like a first date.

PRACTICE OPEN HONESTY

Communication with open honesty takes practice, and it does require both partners to be willing and open to improve those communication skills. If the effort is one-sided, it will be hard to practice. We understand that when you are focused on getting through your days without causing conflict, bringing up the more challenging conversations can feel virtually impossible. The more you practice openly communicating, the easier it will be. We recommend setting aside a safe space and time to have harder conversations with a mutual agreement in place to allow for patience and practice.

ELIMINATE "YOU" STATEMENTS

This is Communication 101 for everyone: Drop "you" and turn to "I" statements.

DRINK A GLASS OF WATER

What? Yes. If you're in the storm of conflict and desperate to retaliate, try to drink a small glass of water and then see how you feel. This can help to temper the fire and create a pause for emotional regulation.

SCHEDULE THERAPY WHEN NEEDED

Don't be afraid of couples therapy if it's needed. Sometimes, a few sessions can help break the communication barrier, and a little bit will go a long way. We understand that this takes time and money (both everyday stressors), so adding therapy on top of that can feel insurmountable. However, don't be overwhelmed in thinking of therapy as a permanent thing. The commitment of going a few times can speak volumes about the value you place on your relationship.

And if you are still wondering why we're going on about communication in a chapter about sex, here's why:

COMMUNICATION DEEPENS TRUST

A trusting relationship creates a safe environment where partners feel comfortable exploring their sexuality, leading to reduced anxiety and enhanced sexual pleasure. Trust builds as we authentically and consistently engage our partners in meaningful communication and conversation.

COMMUNICATION REDUCES STRESS

It's not uncommon to end up feeling like you and your partner are living on separate islands, with limited ability to openly communicate without causing a disruption. Would you rather keep something to yourself than potentially cause a fight? We've been there. A supportive relationship can reduce stress and anxiety, but we understand that this is often not the case. Setting aside time each week to talk about life, goals, dreams, and desires can be a profound way to bridge the communication gap, establish better communication skills, reduce stress, and move beyond the day-to-day chatter.

COMMUNICATION EASES THE BURDEN

Whether you are in a new relationship or a long-term one with family obligations, sharing responsibilities is vital to maintaining a healthy sex life. We speak from the perspective of mothers and women who experience so many of the managerial (and super unsexy) aspects of life falling on us. We recommend speaking up and asking for what you want from your partner. When you need help, be kind, but be direct. We promise you will see the indirect benefits in your overall communication and in your sex life.

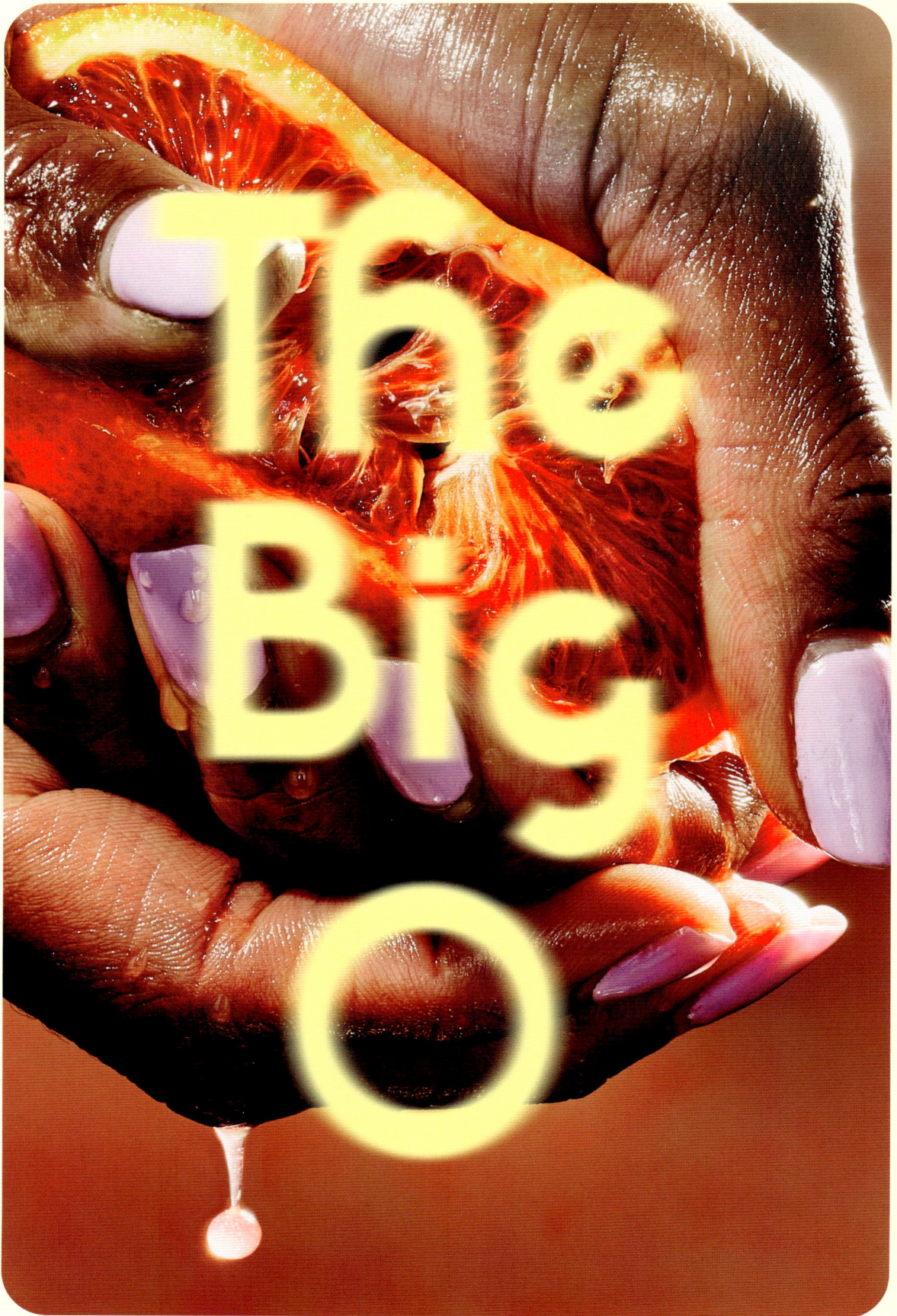

The Big O

The culmination of all aspects of sexual health is the orgasm. Orgasms are celebrated for their intense pleasure and intimacy, but did you know that their benefits extend beyond pure enjoyment? They are also great for our physical health and our mental well-being.

Why does the orgasm exist? And what is its function? →

The biological reasons for orgasm include reproductive function, bonding and intimacy, stress relief, and as a primary motivator for sexual activity. Much like the libido, the orgasm encompasses a combination of physiological processes, brain activity, evolutionary advantages, and psychological benefits, all contributing to the overall experience and importance of orgasm in human life.

Although reaching orgasm can be very different for all genders, the biological aspect is essentially the same—increasing pleasure as a motivating factor for bonding and sometimes as a precursor to procreation.

The list of health benefits of orgasm is long and varied and includes:

STRESS RELIEF

One of the most immediate benefits of orgasm is the ability to reduce stress levels through the release of endorphins, or "feel good" hormones. These endorphins induce the feelings of relaxation and euphoria associated with orgasm. This natural high reduces stress and can improve mood and mental health.

PHYSICAL HEALTH

The physiological responses from orgasm benefit our bodies by increasing blood flow and circulation. This can include better skin health, heart health, and overall improved circulation. For those with uteruses, the physical health aspects include pelvic floor strength and improved vaginal health from wall lubrication and elasticity. In those with penises, regular ejaculation has been associated with a reduced risk of prostate cancer, as it helps flush out potentially harmful substances from the prostate gland.[8]

PAIN RELIEF

The release of endorphins during orgasm not only elevates mood but also serves as a natural painkiller. This effect can alleviate various types of pain, from headaches to menstrual cramps, offering a nonpharmacological alternative for pain management.

IMMUNE SYSTEM BOOST

Studies suggest that orgasms may strengthen the immune system in some capacity. The surge of cortisol during sexual arousal, followed by the release of endorphins and other neurotransmitters, can enhance immune functions, helping the body better defend against infections.[9]

IMPROVED SLEEP

Studies show that orgasms may promote better sleep patterns or the perception of better sleep. All genders reported improved sleep quality and reduced sleep latency when sex with a partner involved an orgasm, with no significant differences between genders. These results support the hypothesis that higher levels of oxytocin and prolactin after orgasm can facilitate better sleep.[10]

MENTAL WELL-BEING

Orgasms release feel-good neurochemicals like dopamine and oxytocin that boost your satisfaction, which may lead to increased happiness and better mental health. This can also reduce symptoms of anxiety and depression by promoting a sense of well-being and connection.

LONGEVITY

Research suggests weak but positive associations between the enjoyment of sexual activity and longevity. However, this association was stronger among individuals who consider sexuality to be necessary and less significant to those who do not consider sexuality as an essential lifestyle factor. The combined benefits of reduced stress, enhanced cardiovascular health, and improved immune function may contribute to the positive association.[11]

Orgasms are moments of pleasure and can be essential to our overall health, well-being, and satisfaction. They offer many physical, emotional, and psychological benefits that enhance our lives. Recognizing and appreciating these positive impacts can contribute to a healthier and more fulfilling lifestyle.

203

How to Have More (and Better) Sex— According to Science

Sexual intimacy and science may not feel like a natural fit for most of us. When you're talking about sex, the last thing you want to think about is the science behind it. But understanding why, how, and what's behind how it all works can be a very important aspect of improving your sex life—because, let's be honest, sex education for most of us was severely lacking in quality content.

Proper sex education empowers individuals to enhance both their physical and mental well-being, leading to higher-quality and more satisfying sexual experiences. By understanding the physiological and psychological factors involved in sexual activity, people can improve communication with their partners, address potential sexual dysfunctions, and make informed decisions about their sexual health. This knowledge also fosters greater confidence, reduces anxiety, and helps build stronger, more intimate relationships. Ultimately, understanding the science of sex allows individuals to take control of their sexual health, promoting overall well-being and a more positive approach to sexual experiences.

STEP 1: COMMUNICATION AND CONNECTION ARE PRIORITIES

We've already laid out the importance of quality communication, and it is substantial. Effective communication and emotional connection are crucial for a satisfying sexual relationship. Communication about desires, boundaries, and emotional needs fosters trust and intimacy.

Setting aside time to communicate is the first step to successful communication, and it needs to be something that both partners enjoy or look forward to. While "date night" is always an option to get communication started, we believe it needs to become more of a daily or biweekly habit.

STEP 2: MAINTAIN PHYSICAL AND MENTAL HEALTH

Easier said than done, and always a priority for many reasons, but if mental and physical health is suffering in one partner (or both), it is virtually impossible to meet each other's needs. Better physical health = better sex, and that's a given. Regular exercise promotes cardiovascular fitness, boosts mood, and increases neurotransmitters such as dopamine and serotonin, which boost pleasure and happiness.

STEP 3: SCHEDULE QUALITY TIME TOGETHER

"When I first suggested 'scheduled quality time' to my husband, he cringed. It sounds super unsexy, operational, and like forced fun. But if you want quality time, you've got to schedule it!" —MEREDITH

Unfortunately, scheduling is the key to getting anything done, including quality time, for most of us who work and manage family life. So, get over it and just do it.

STEP 4: CHANGE THE SCENERY

Novelty and new experiences stimulate the brain's reward system to increase dopamine, leading to increased pleasure and satisfaction. New techniques, positions, or settings all lead to reports of higher levels of sexual fulfillment and relationship satisfaction.

STEP 5: ADDRESS POTENTIAL BARRIERS

Identify what is getting in the way of having better, more satisfying sex. Whether it's physical health, mental stress, or simply not having enough time, you must be willing to look at and address potential barriers to sexual intimacy. Research-based approaches to stress management (see Chapter 6: Help Your Self Stress Less, page 168), mindfulness, and medical interventions can improve libido and sexual function, promoting a healthier and more satisfying sex life.

SEXUAL
HEALTH IS
ABOUT
VITALITY

205

It's about an energy that extends far beyond our mainstream vision of what's "sexy," or the physical act of sex. If you are not feeling lit up in your life or your relationships, tapping into that energy can be difficult if not impossible. We hope this chapter helps you understand the psychological and physiological aspects of sexual health, and how sexual health affects your overall sense of health and well-being. Knowledge is power, and armed with this information, we hope you can find that spark within.

The Recipes

We eat with our eyes first, and while there are many ingredients that have vitamins and minerals to promote sexual health, most of the foods we associate with better sex often have a visual component that serves as innuendo. Sexy-looking, as a means to being good for sex.

Although none of the recipes in this chapter are hard to make, they do feel slightly special-occasion and would be great served as a special-occasion meal. And, of course, there is chocolate . . .

→ **Beet Carpaccio**

→ **Lion's Mane Tacos**

→ **Dark Chocolate Truffles**

Beet Carpaccio, Almond Ricotta, and Herbs

Beet carpaccio is one of those dishes that is easier than you'd think to make but has such a big visual impact. If you can get your hands on some candy cane beets you will automatically have a dish that looks especially "fancy." You can present the carpaccio on a platter with dollops of almond ricotta, or assemble into ricotta-filled beet "ravioli" utilizing the same ingredients.

Almond ricotta is easy enough to make but does require some prep time. If you don't have the patience, there are definitely some high-quality nondairy alternatives on the market that would be an easy substitute.

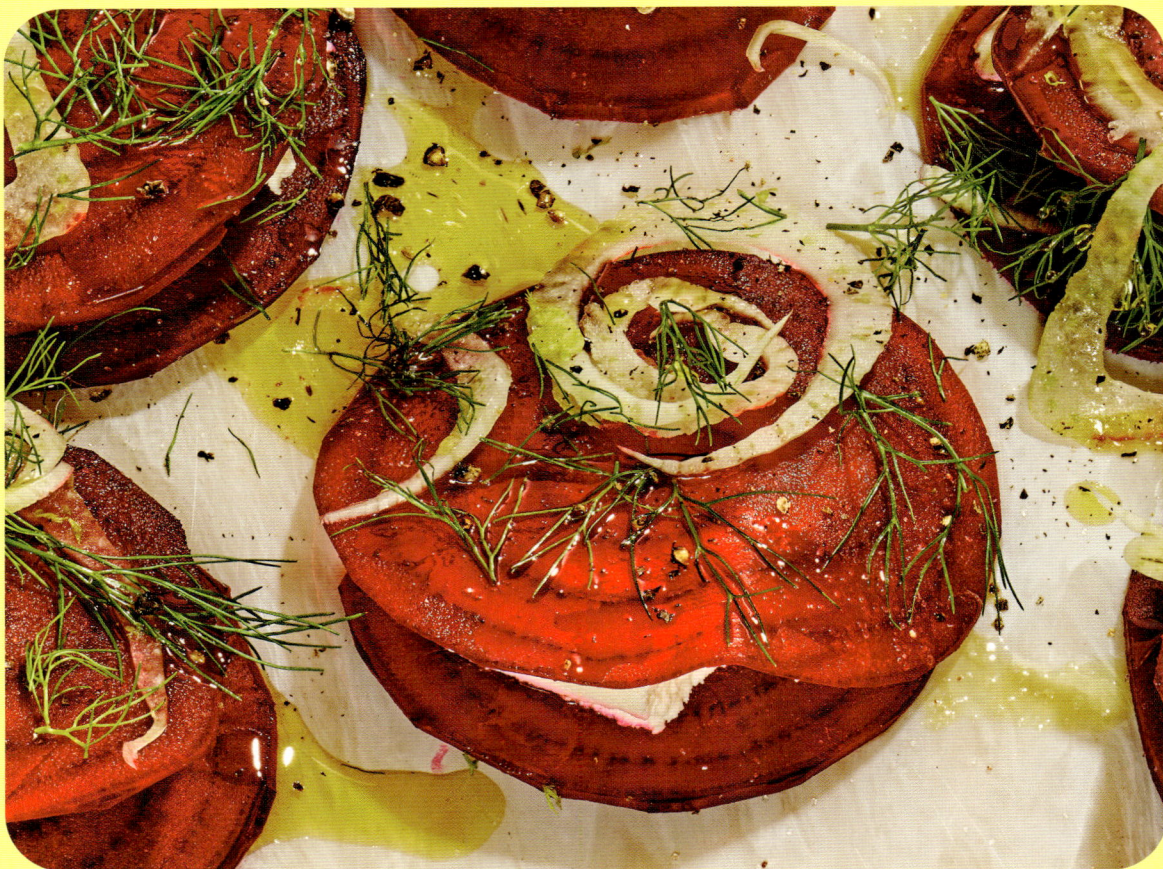

SERVES 4

**FOR THE BEET
CARPACCIO:**
3 medium-size beets. Red,
yellow, and candy cane
varieties are all beautiful!

2 tablespoons olive oil

1 tablespoon fresh lemon
juice

1 teaspoon sea salt

1 tablespoon balsamic
vinegar

Salt and freshly ground
black pepper

**FOR THE ALMOND
RICOTTA:**
1 cup (120 g) blanched
almonds, soaked in water
overnight

2 tablespoons nutritional
yeast

1 clove garlic, minced

2 tablespoons fresh lemon
juice

3 tablespoons olive oil

1 teaspoon white miso

FOR GARNISH:
Mint, basil, parsley, or
mixed microgreens

Chopped pistachios or
almonds (optional)

2 tablespoons capers,
drained (optional)

Extra-virgin olive oil, for
drizzling

Salt and freshly ground
black pepper

How to make?

→ Make the beets

Peel the beets and thinly slice them using a mandoline or a sharp
knife. They should be as close to paper-thin as possible.

In a bowl, gently toss the beets with olive oil, lemon juice, sea salt,
and vinegar and allow to marinate for at least 30 minutes.

→ Make the almond ricotta

Drain and rinse the soaked almonds. In a food processor, combine
the almonds, nutritional yeast, garlic, lemon juice, olive oil, salt,
and pepper.

Process until smooth but still fluffy and creamy; do not over-blend.
You can make the ricotta ahead of time as it will keep in an airtight
container in the refrigerator for up to 4 days.

→ To present a platter of carpaccio

Shingle-layer the beet slices on a medium to large serving platter.
Dollop the ricotta over the beet slices.

Drizzle with olive oil and sprinkle with the herbs and the capers, if
using. Season with salt and pepper.

Finish with the chopped nuts, if using.

→ Tip

You can purchase blanched almonds, but we like to blanch our
own. Just bring a small pot of water to a boil, add 1 cup (120 g) raw
almonds to the pot, and let them boil for about 60 seconds (no
more, or they will get too soft!). Rinse immediately with cold water.
The skins will come off easily at this point.

VARIATION—BEET "RAVIOLI":
Layer one beet slice, 1 tablespoon of ricotta, topped with another
beet slice to resemble ravioli.

Garnish with herbs, nuts, and capers, if using, drizzle with olive oil,
and season with salt and pepper.

209

Lion's Mane Tacos
with Lime Crema

SERVES 4

1 pound (455 g) lion's mane mushrooms

2 tablespoons olive or avocado oil

2 cloves garlic, minced

1 teaspoon ground cumin

1 teaspoon smoked paprika

½ teaspoon chili powder

1 tablespoon tamari or nama shoyu

Salt and freshly ground black pepper

½ teaspoon cayenne pepper (optional)

¼ cup (60 ml) water or stock

½ medium onion, diced

Fresh cilantro, roughly chopped

Corn tortillas (we love blue corn tortillas)

1 recipe Lime Crema (recipe follows)

Toppings of your choice, such as sliced avocado, chopped tomato, and lettuce leaves

Lion's mane is becoming more readily available in grocery stores, and if you see it, we highly recommend trying it, as it is an excellent meat substitute. If you can't find lion's mane, then oyster mushrooms can be substituted in the same preparation.

How to make?

Clean the mushrooms by gently wiping them with a damp cloth. You don't want to wet them as it will change the texture. Tear them into pieces resembling meat. (Lion's mane has a great texture for mimicking shredded pork.)

Heat the oil in a large skillet over medium heat. Add the garlic and sauté for about 1 minute until fragrant.

Add the mushrooms to the skillet and sauté for 5 to 7 minutes, until they start to soften and brown slightly. Season the mushrooms with the cumin, smoked paprika, chili powder, tamari, and a pinch each of salt and pepper. Stir in the cayenne (if using).

Add the water (a few tablespoons at a time) to finish the sauté and deglaze the pan, scraping up any bits from the bottom of the skillet.

Continue to cook for about 5 minutes more, until the mushrooms are tender and have absorbed any water and the flavors. Taste and adjust for salt and heat and remove the pan from the heat.

To assemble the tacos, warm the tortillas in a dry skillet or on a griddle until pliable.

Spread about 1 tablespoon of lime crema on each tortilla and add the toppings of your choice.

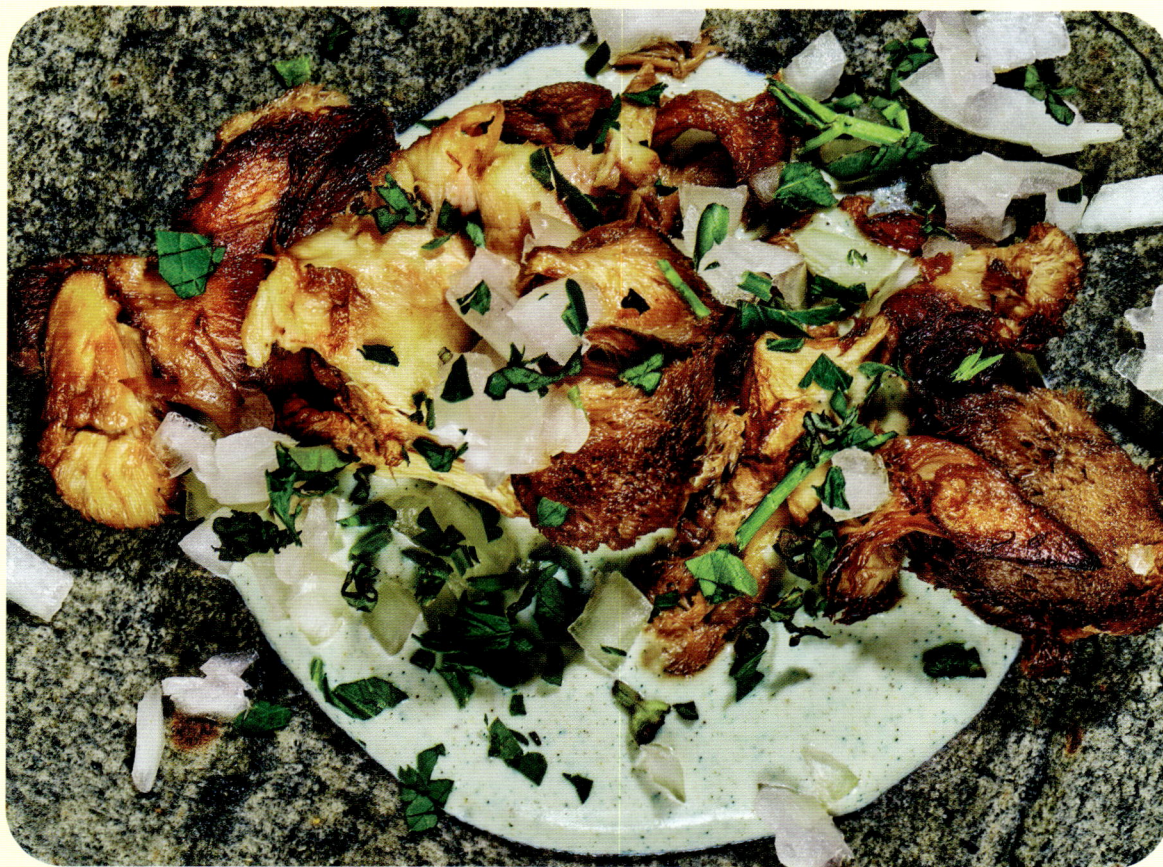

Lime Crema

MAKES ABOUT 1.5 CUPS (360 ML)

1 cup (130 g) cashews, soaked in water for at least 4 hours if not using a high-speed blender

Juice of 1 lime

1 tablespoon nutritional yeast (optional)

½ teaspoon salt

1 clove garlic, roughly chopped

¼ teaspoon onion powder

1 teaspoon ground coriander or a small handful of fresh cilantro leaves or stems (optional)

How to make?

NOTE
Soaking the cashews in water until softened is not necessary if using a high-speed blender, but is recommended if you aren't.

To a blender, add ½ cup (65 g) cashews, ½ cup (120 ml) water, the lime juice, nutritional yeast (if using), salt, garlic, and onion powder. Blend until smooth and creamy.

Taste and adjust the seasonings accordingly. You could whisk in the coriander, or a small handful of fresh cilantro for extra flavor.

If the cream is too thick, add more water, a tablespoon at a time, until you reach your desired consistency.

Serve with anything from tacos to nachos or as a salad dressing.

Keeps in an airtight container in the refrigerator for up to 5 days.

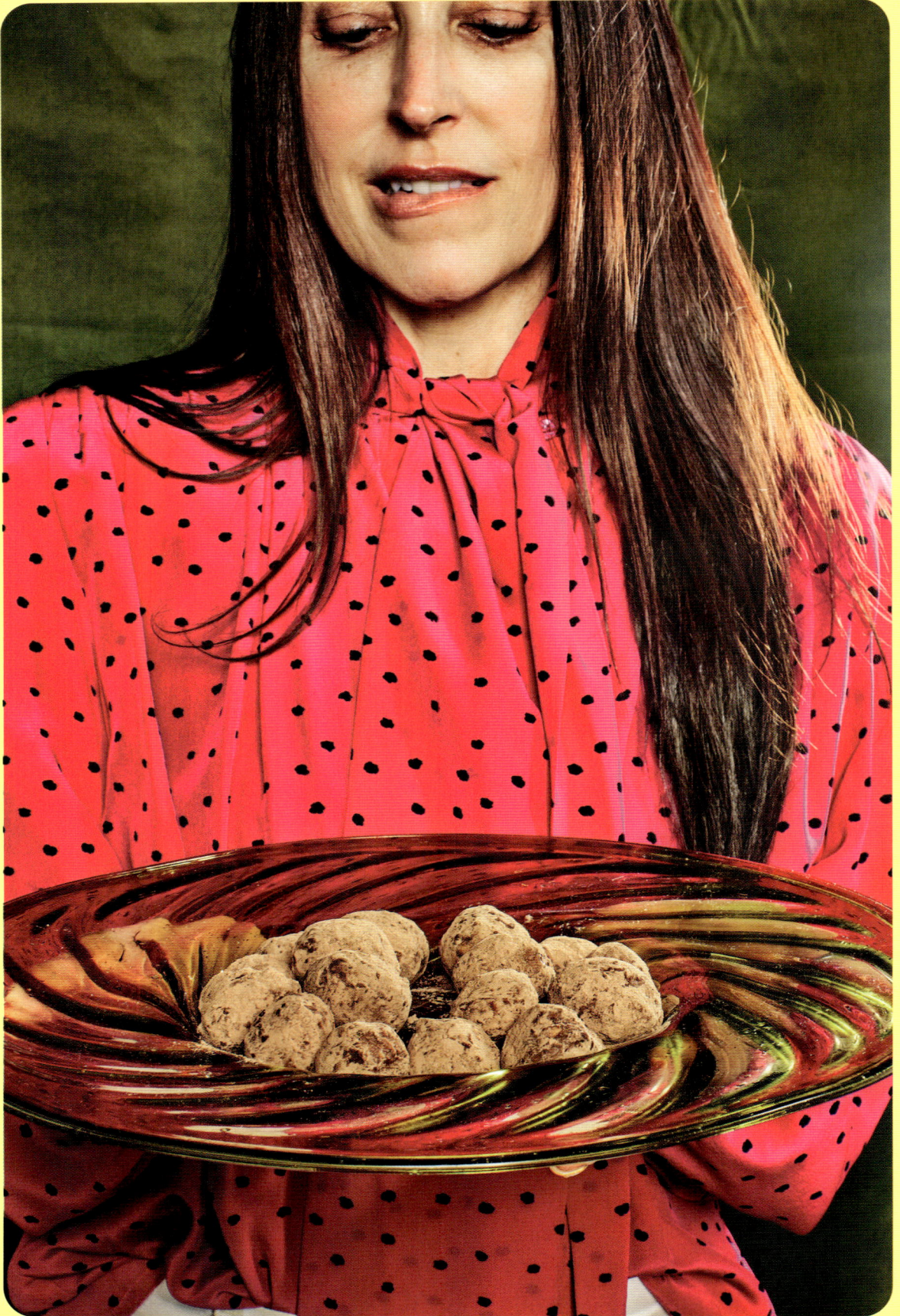

The Darkest Dark Chocolate Truffles

(with Optional Maca)

Chocolate truffles are one of the easiest high-impact desserts you can make. Everyone loves them, and they literally take 30 minutes to make.

Maca is a hero ingredient in this recipe, if you include it. It is a root native to the Andes mountains that is known for its hormone-balancing properties, and the balance it offers may help to naturally enhance sex drive and increase fertility. It's backed by a long history of use, and by science!

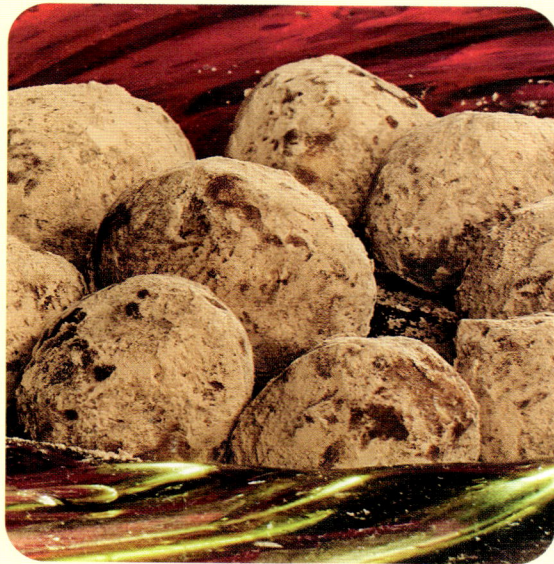

**MAKES ABOUT
12 TRUFFLES**

1 cup (95 g) cacao powder

¾ cup (180 ml) maple syrup

1 tablespoon maca powder (optional)

1 teaspoon pure vanilla extract

½ teaspoon sea salt

2 tablespoons almond or cashew butter

Pinch ground cinnamon (optional)

½ cup (120 ml) coconut oil, melted

½ cup (120 ml) cacao butter, melted (sub coconut oil if necessary)

¼ cup (30 g) cacao nibs, cacao powder, coconut flakes, or chopped nuts, for coating

How to make?

In a high-speed blender, add the cacao powder, maple syrup, maca powder (if using), vanilla, sea salt, almond butter, and cinnamon (if using) and blend until smooth. Slowly add the coconut oil and cacao butter and continue to blend until silky smooth. Pour into a bowl and refrigerate for about 5 minutes (not longer!), until the truffe batter is firm enough to mold. (You want it to be about the texture of cookie dough.)

Using a tablespoon, scoop up one truffle at a time and roll the batter in your hands to create a 1½-inch (4 cm) ball. Refrigerate for about 15 minutes before serving. If coating in a garnish, pour the topping of your choice into a small bowl and roll the truffles in the cacao nibs, cacao powder, coconut flakes, or chopped nuts before serving.

The truffles keep for up to 2 months in an airtight container in the refrigerator.

CONCLUSION

Help Your Self. We hope this book empowers you with the understanding that health thrives on rhythms and routines. Our bodies function best when their natural cycles are supported, allowing everything to work harmoniously without unnecessary interference.

The force-it-to-fix mentalities that many of us gravitate toward do not support holistic health. Extreme diets, intense routines, rigid restrictions, and an "all-or-nothing" approach are not the foundation for sustainable well-being. Too often, wellness culture promotes these extremes and hyper-fixations, but the truth is, they don't align with how most of us live—or how we're meant to thrive in a balanced way.

We also understand that health looks different for everyone. Some of the practices shared here might feel easy to integrate into your life, while others may take more time or feel less relevant to your circumstances. That's okay. This book isn't about perfection or fear; it's about finding what works for you and creating space for wellness in a way that feels achievable and supportive.

Ultimately, our goal is to help you build a foundation for health that feels steady, nourishing, and aligned with your life. Small, consistent steps and an approach rooted in balance can lead to meaningful, lasting change. We're so glad you're here and hope this journey brings you clarity, empowerment, and enjoyment!

ACKNOWLEDGMENTS

This project would not have been possible without the enthusiasm and support of so many incredible individuals. We are so grateful.

Erinn Glynn, PhD, our dedicated researcher, you went above and beyond in pulling together the details and information we needed to make this project shine. Your work was truly amazing, and we couldn't have done this without you.

Heami Lee, our brilliant photographer, you brought this vision to life with your incredible talent and energy. You made the process not only seamless but genuinely fun in every way. And to Ashley Butts, your support as photography assistant was invaluable—thank you for your positivity and professionalism.

To Eileen O'Dea of the Wooden Palate, your artistry and impeccable eye as our prop stylist elevated every photo. Jessica Sindler, our sharp and thoughtful developmental editor, thank you for helping us polish this work and truly kick it up a notch. Your keen attention to detail made all the difference.

And from Meredith . . .

To my husband and daughter, my constant sources of motivation, inspiration, and mostly enthusiastic recipe testers. I love you both so much.

To Kat—your vision, passion, and ability to make things happen have been a huge inspiration to me. I am so grateful that we met.

To everyone who contributed to this journey, thank you from the bottom of my heart. This work is a reflection of your collective talent and spirit, and I am so honored to have had the chance to collaborate with all of you.

From Kat . . .

My three little girls, Tali, Mika, and Sofi, you are my heart and the reason this book got started for me, as I aspire to build the healthiest life for you all. To my husband, who first read this book and said, *Wow, this sounds like everything you tell me to do and how to live*. I love you for keeping me balanced so I don't go off into the deep end of science and wellness.

To Meredith, I'm so glad we met before we started our businesses. I'm continually inspired by your hard work and passion for food and better living. Also your moderate approach to doing what feels good.

To my team at Ritual: Lindsay, Nima, and Mastaneh, I've learned so much from you!

Finally, I want to thank my mom, Faina, who battled cancer and practiced macrobiotics. You've inspired me for decades to be curious about medicine, science, and nutrition.

Notes

CHAPTER 1 HELP YOUR SELF GET STARTED

1. A. D. Termannsen, K. K. B. Clemmensen, J. M. Thomsen, et al., "Effects of vegan diets on cardiometabolic health: A systematic review and meta-analysis of randomized controlled trials," *Obesity Review* 23, no. 9 (September 2022): e13462. doi: 10.1111/obr.13462.

2. J. S. Dybvik, M. Svendsen, and D. Aune, "Vegetarian and vegan diets and the risk of cardiovascular disease, ischemic heart disease and stroke: a systematic review and meta-analysis of prospective cohort studies," *European Journal of Nutrition* 62, no. 1 (February 2023): 51–69. doi: 10.1007/s00394-022-02942-8.

3. T. Huang, B. Yang, J. Zheng, et al., "Cardiovascular disease mortality and cancer incidence in vegetarians: A meta-analysis and systematic review," *Annals of Nutrition and Metabolism* 60, no. 4 (2012): 233–40.

4. S. Tonstad , T. Butler, R. Yan, et al., "Type of vegetarian diet, body weight, and prevalence of Type 2 diabetes," *Diabetes Care* 32, no. 5 (May 2009): 791–966. doi: 10.2337/dc08-1886.

5. T. Huang, B. Yang, J. Zheng, et al. "Cardiovascular disease mortality and cancer incidence in vegetarians: A meta-analysis and systematic review." *Annals of Nutrition and Metabolism* 60, no. 4 (2012):233-40. doi: 10.1159/000337301.

6. Huang et al., "Cardiovascular disease mortality and cancer incidence in vegetarians."

7. S. Langyan, P. Yadava, F. N. Khan, et al., "Sustaining Protein Nutrition Through Plant-Based Foods," *Frontiers in Nutrition* 8 (January 2022): 772573. doi: 10.3389/fnut.2021.772573.

8. D. R. Jacobs, Jr., E. H. Haddad, A. J. Lanou, et al., "Food, plant food, and vegetarian diets in the US dietary guidelines: Conclusions of an expert panel," *American Journal of Clinical Nutrition* 89, no. 5 (May 2009): 1549S–1552S. https://doi.org/10.3945/ajcn.2009.26736C.

9. K. E. Reed, J. Camargo, J. Hamilton-Reeves, et al., "Neither soy nor isoflavone intake affects male reproductive hormones: An expanded and updated meta-analysis of clinical studies," *Reproductive Toxicology* 100 (March 2021): 60–67. doi: 10.1016/j.reprotox.2020.12.019.

10. M. Messina, A. Duncan, V. Messina, et al., "The health effects of soy: A reference guide for health professionals," *Frontiers in Nutrition* 11, no. 9 (August 2022): 970364. doi: 10.3389/fnut.2022.970364.

11. A. P. Simopoulos, "The importance of the ratio of omega-6/omega-3 essential fatty acids," *Biomedical Pharmacotherapy* 56, no. 8 (October 2002): 365–79. doi: 10.1016/s0753-3322(02)00253-6.

12. Nurhan Dunford, "Oil and Oilseed Processing II," Oklahoma State University, July 1, 2016, https://extension.okstate.edu/fact-sheets/oil-and-oilseed-processing-ii.html.

13. "Fats and oils in human nutrition: Report of a joint expert consultation, Food and Agriculture Organization of the United Nations and the World Health Organization," *FAO Food Nutrition Papers* 57 (1994): i–xix, 1–147.

14. C. Y. Ng, X. F. Leong, N. Masbah, et al., "Heated vegetable oils and cardiovascular disease risk factors" (reprint), *Vascular Pharmacology* 62, no. 1 (July 2014): 38–46. doi: 10.1016/j.vph.2014.05.003.

CHAPTER 2 HELP YOUR SELF LOVE YOUR GUT

1. "Probiotics and Prebiotics," World Gastroenterology Organisation Global Guidelines, https://www.worldgastroenterology.org/UserFiles/file/guidelines/probiotics-and-prebiotics-english-2017.pdf.

2. P. J. Turnbaugh, M. Hamady, T. Yatsunenko, et al., "A core gut microbiome in obese and lean twins," *Nature* 457, no. 7228 (January 22, 2009):480–84. doi: 10.1038/nature07540.

3. P. Li, X. Chang, X. Chen, et al., "Early-life antibiotic exposure increases the risk of childhood overweight and obesity in relation to dysbiosis of gut microbiota: a birth cohort study," *Annals of Clinical Microbiology and Antimicrobials* 21, no. 1 (November 3, 2022): 46.

4. T. P. Van Boeckel, C. Brower, M. Gilbert, et al., "Global trends in antimicrobial use in food animals," *Proceedings of the National Academy of Sciences* 112, no. 18 (March 19, 2015): 5649–54. https://doi.org/10.1073/pnas.1503141112.

5. N. T. Mueller, M. K. Differding, H. Sun, et al., "Maternal Bacterial Engraftment in Multiple Body

Sites of Cesarean Section Born Neonates after Vaginal Seeding: A Randomized Controlled Trial," *mBio* 14, no. 3 (June 27, 2023): e0049123. doi: 10.1128/mbio.00491-23.

6. Z.-W. Guan, E.-Z. Yu, Q. Feng, "Soluble Dietary Fiber, One of the Most Important Nutrients for the Gut Microbiota," *Molecules* 26 (2021): 6802. https://doi.org/10.3390/molecules26226802.

7. G. Riccardi and A. A. Rivellese, "Effects of dietary fiber and carbohydrate on glucose and lipoprotein metabolism in diabetic patients," *Diabetes Care* 14, no. 12 (December 1991): 1115–25. doi: 10.2337/diacare.14.12.1115.

8. Johnson W. McRorie, Jr., and Nicola M. McKeown, "Understanding the Physics of Functional Fibers in the Gastrointestinal Tract: An Evidence-Based Approach to Resolving Enduring Misconceptions about Insoluble and Soluble Fiber," *Journal of the Academy of Nutrition and Dietetics* 117, no. 2: 251–64.

9. T. Dinan, Y. Borre, and J. Cryan, "Genomics of schizophrenia: time to consider the gut microbiome?," **Molecular Psychiatry** 19 (2014): 1252–57. https://doi.org/10.1038/mp.2014.93

10. A. Del Colle, N. Israelyan, K. Gross Margolis, "Novel aspects of enteric serotonergic signaling in health and brain-gut disease," *American Journal of Physiology-Gastrointestinal and Liver Physiology* 318, no. 1 (January 1, 2020): G130–G143. doi: 10.1152/ajpgi.00173.2019.

11. F. Donoso, J. F. Cryan, L. Olavarría-Ramírez, "Inflammation, Lifestyle Factors, and the Microbiome-Gut-Brain Axis: Relevance to Depression and Antidepressant Action," *Clinical Pharmacology & Therapeutics* 113, no. 2 (February 2023): 246–59. doi: 10.1002/cpt.2581.

12. S. Breit, A. Kupferberg, G. Rogler, et al., "Vagus Nerve as Modulator of the Brain-Gut Axis in Psychiatric and Inflammatory Disorders," Frontiers in Psychiatry (March 13, 2018): 44. doi: 10.3389/fpsyt.2018.00044.

13. K. Suzuki, C. N. Jayasena, S. R. Bloom, "The gut hormones in appetite regulation," *Journal of Obesity* (2011): 528401. doi: 10.1155/2011/528401.

14. K. Kasarello, A. Cudnoch-Jedrzejewska, K. Czarzasta, "Communication of gut microbiota and brain via immune and neuroendocrine signaling," *Frontiers in Microbiology* (January 25, 2023): 1118529. doi: 10.3389/fmicb.2023.1118529.

15. Glenn R. Gibson and Marcel B. Roberfroid, "Dietary Modulation of the Human Colonic Microbiota: Introducing the Concept of Prebiotics," Journal of Nutrition 125, no. 6 (1995): 1401–12. https://doi.org/10.1093/jn/125.6.1401.

16. M. Roberfroid, G. R. Gibson, L. Hoyles, et al., "Prebiotic effects: Metabolic and health benefits," British Journal of Nutrition 104 (August 2010): S1–63. doi: 10.1017/S0007114510003363.

17. Gibson and Roberfroid, "Dietary Modulation of the Human Colonic Microbiota."

18. C. A. M. Wegh, S. Y. Geerlings, J. Knol, et al., "Postbiotics and Their Potential Applications in Early Life Nutrition and Beyond," International Journal of Molecular Sciences 20, no. 19 (September 20, 2019): 4673. doi: 10.3390/ijms20194673.

CHAPTER 3 HELP YOUR SELF AGE WELL

1. David J. Hunter, "For Disease Risk, Is It Genes or the Environment? Probably Both," Harvard T. H. Chan School of Public Health, December 14, 2018.

2. A. Hajialiasgary Najafabadi, M. H. Soheilifar, and N. Masoudi-Khoram, "Exosomes in skin photoaging: Biological functions and therapeutic opportunity," *Cell Communication and Signaling* 22, no. 32 (2024). https://doi.org/10.1186/s12964-023-01451-3.

3. Y. Hong, A. Boiti, D. Vallone, et al., "Reactive Oxygen Species Signaling and Oxidative Stress: Transcriptional Regulation and Evolution," *Antioxidants* 13 (2024): 312. https://doi.org/10.3390/antiox13030312.

4. Hajialiasgary Najafabadi et al., "Exosomes in skin photoaging."

5. S. Q. Wang, Y. Balagula, and U. Osterwalder, "Photoprotection: A Review of the Current and Future Technologies," *Dermatologic Therapy* (January–February 2010): 31–47. https://doi.org/10.1111/j.1529-8019.2009.01289.x

6. Wang et al., "Photoprotection."

7. A. Fourtanier, D. Moyal, and S. Seite, "Sunscreens containing the broad-spectrum UVA absorber, Mexoryl® SX, prevent the cutaneous detrimental effects of UV exposure: A review of clinical study results," *Photodermatology, Photoimmunology & Photomedicine* 24, no. 4 (August 2008): 164–74. https://doi.org/10.1111/j.1600-0781.2008.00365.

8. B. Herzog, M. Wehrle, and K. Quass, "Photostability of UV absorber systems in sunscreens," *Photochemistry and Photobiology* 85, no. 4 (July–August 2009): 869–78. doi: 10.1111/j.1751-1097.2009.00544.x.

9. C. G. Hayden, M. S. Roberts, and H. A. Benson, "Systemic absorption of sunscreen after topical application," *Lancet* 350, no. 9081 (September 20, 1997): 863–64. doi: 10.1016/S0140-6736(05)62032-6.

10. D. Darr, S. Combs, S. Dunston, et al., "Topical vitamin C protects porcine skin from ultraviolet radiation-induced damage," *British Journal of Dermatology* 127, no. 3, (September 1, 1992): 247–53. https://doi.org/10.1111/j.1365-2133.1992.tb00122.x.

11. S. Mukherjee, A. Date, V. Patravale, et al., "Retinoids in the treatment of skin aging: An overview of clinical efficacy and safety," *Clinical Interventions in Aging* 1, no. 4 (2006): 327–48. doi: 10.2147/ciia.2006.1.4.327.

12. J. M. Pullar, A. C. Carr, and M. C. M. Vissers, "The Roles of Vitamin C in Skin Health," *Nutrients* 9, no. 8 (August 12, 2017): 866. doi: 10.3390/nu9080866.

13. J. Levin and S. B. Momin, "How much do we really know about our favorite cosmeceutical ingredients?," Journal of Clinical and Aesthetic Dermatology 3, no. 2 (February 2010): 22–41.

14. M. Ash, M. Zibitt, O. Shauly, et al., "The Innovative and Evolving Landscape of Topical Exosome and Peptide Therapies: A Systematic Review of the Available Literature," *Aesthetic Surgery Journal Open Forum* 6 (March 19, 2024): ojae017. doi: 10.1093/asjof/ojae017.

15. M. Essendoubi, C. Gobinet, R. Reynaud, et al., "Human skin penetration of hyaluronic acid of different molecular weights as probed by Raman spectroscopy," Skin Research and Technology 22, no. 1 (February 2016): 55–62. doi: 10.1111/srt.12228.

16. T. K. Leo, E. S. S. Tan, F. Amini, et al., "Effect of Rice (Oryza sativa L.) Ceramides Supplementation on Improving Skin Barrier Functions and Depigmentation: An Open-Label Prospective Study," *Nutrients* 14, no. 13 (June 30, 2022): 2737. doi: 10.3390/nu14132737.

17. E. Proksch, M. Schunck, V. Zague, "Oral intake of specific bioactive collagen peptides reduces skin wrinkles and increases dermal matrix synthesis," *Skin Pharmacology and Physiology* 27, no. 3 (2014): 113–19. doi: 10.1159/000355523.

18. R. Katta and D. N. Brown, "Diet and Skin Cancer: The Potential Role of Dietary Antioxidants in Nonmelanoma Skin Cancer Prevention," *Journal of Skin Cancer* (2015): 893149. doi: 10.1155/2015/893149.

19. "The Science of Gua Sha," Pacific College of Health and Science, May 5, 2015, https://www.pacificcollege.edu/news/press-releases/2015/05/05/the-science-of-gua-sha.

20. K. Armstrong, R. Gokal, A. Chevalier, et al., "Microcurrent Point Stimulation Applied to Lower Back Acupuncture Points for the Treatment of Nonspecific Neck Pain," *Journal of Alternative and Complementary Medicine* 23, no. 4 (April 2017): 295–99. doi: 10.1089/acm.2016.0313.

21. P. Bu, R. Duan, J. Luo, et al., "Development of Home Beauty Devices for Facial Rejuvenation: Establishment of Efficacy Evaluation System," *Clinical, Cosmetic and Investigational Dermatology* 17 (March 8, 2024): 553–63. doi: 10.2147/CCID.S449599.

22. Bu et al., "Development of Home Beauty Devices."

23. A. Singh and S. Yadav, "Microneedling: Advances and widening horizons," *Indian Dermatology Online Journal* 7, no. 4 (July–August 2016): 244-54. doi: 10.4103/2229-5178.185468.

CHAPTER 4 HELP YOUR SELF HYDRATE

1. B. M. Popkin, K. E. D'Anci, and I. H. Rosenberg, "Water, hydration, and health," *Nutrition Reviews* 68, no. 8 (August 2010): 439–58. doi: 10.1111/j.1753-4887.2010.00304.x.

2. A. Adan, "Cognitive performance and dehydration," *Journal of the American College of Nutrition* 31, no. 2 (April 2012): 71–78. doi: 10.1080/07315724.2012.10720011.

3. L. E. Armstrong, M. S. Ganio, D. J. Casa, et al., "Mild dehydration affects mood in healthy young women," *Journal of Nutrition* 142, no. 2 (February 2012): 382–88. doi: 10.3945/jn.111.142000.

4. W. F. Clark, J. M. Sontrop, J. J. Macnab, et al., "Urine volume and change in estimated GFR in a community-based cohort study," *Clinical Journal of the American Society of Nephrology* 6, no. 11 (November 2011): 2634–41. doi: 10.2215/CJN.01990211.

5. D. C. Nieman, "Influence of carbohydrate on the immune response to intensive, prolonged exercise," *Exercise Immunology Review* 4 (1998): 64–76.

6. E. Proksch, J. M. Brandner, J. M. Jensen, "The skin: An indispensable barrier," *Experimental Dermatology* 17, no. 12 (December 2008): 1063–72. doi: 10.1111/j.1600-0625.2008.00786.x.

7. M. Ramos-e-Silva, L. R. Celem, S. Ramos-e-Silva, et al., "Anti-aging cosmetics: Facts and controversies," *Clinics in Dermatology* 28, no. 5 (2010): 565–72.

8. S. M. Shirreffs and R. J. Maughan, "Rehydration and recovery of fluid balance after exercise," *Exercise and Sport Sciences Reviews* 28, no. 1 (January 2000): 27–32.

9. Institute of Medicine, *Dietary Reference Intakes for Water, Potassium, Sodium, Chloride, and Sulfate* (Washington, DC: The National Academies Press, 2005), 77.

10. L. W. Judge, D. M. Bellar, J. K. Popp, et al., "Hydration to Maximize Performance and Recovery: Knowledge, Attitudes, and Behaviors Among Collegiate Track and Field Throwers," *Journal of Human Kinetics* 79 (July 28, 2021):111–22. doi: 10.2478/hukin-2021-0065.

11. "Scientific Opinion on Dietary Reference Values for Water," *European Food Safety Authority Journal* 8, no. 3 (March 25, 2010); Institute of Medicine, *Dietary Reference Intakes*, 77; and "Nordic Council of Ministers Nordic Nutrition Recommendations 2012: Integrating nutrition and physical activity," in *Nordic Nutrition Recommendations. Report No: 5* (Copenhagen: Nordic Council of Ministers), doi: 10.6027/Nord2014-002.

12. Institute of Medicine, *Dietary Reference Intakes*, 77.

13. "In Brief: How Does the Stomach Work?," Institute for Quality and Efficiency in Health Care (IQWiG), Cologne, Germany, 2006–, updated August 5, 2024.

14. D. K. Todd and L. W. Mays, *Groundwater Hydrology*, 3rd ed. (Wiley, 2005).

15. National Research Council (US) Safe Drinking Water Committee, "The Contribution of Drinking Water to Mineral Nutrition in Humans," in *Drinking Water and Health* vol. 3 (Washington, DC: National Academies Press, 1980), https://www.ncbi.nlm.nih.gov/books/NBK216589/.

16. J. J. Foxe, K. P. Morie, P. J. Laud, et al., "Assessing the effects of caffeine and theanine on the maintenance of vigilance during a sustained attention task," *Neuropharmacology* 62, no. 7 (June 2012): 2320–27. doi: 10.1016/j.neuropharm.2012.01.020.

CHAPTER 5 HELP YOUR SELF SLEEP SO GOOD

1. "Circadian Rhythms," National Institute of General Medical Sciences, U.S. Department of Health and Human Services, 2022.

2. "Circadian Rhythms and Circadian Clock," Centers for Disease Control and Prevention, April 1, 2020.

3. "How Sleep Works," National Heart Lung and Blood Institute, U.S. Department of Health and Human Services, 2022.

4. "Brain Basics: Understanding Sleep," National Institute of Neurological Disorders and Stroke, U.S. Department of Health and Human Services, n.d., accessed July 5, 2022.

5. A. K. Patel, V. Reddy, K. R. Shumway, et al., "Physiology, Sleep Stages," *StatPearls*, updated January 26, 2024, https://www.ncbi.nlm.nih.gov/sites/books/NBK526132/.

6. K. Ramar, R. K. Malhotra, K. A. Carden, et al., "Sleep is essential to health: an American Academy of Sleep Medicine position statement," *Journal of Clinical Sleep Medicine* 17, no. 10 (2021): 2115–19.

7. S. Mukherjee, S. R. Patel, S. N. Kales, et al., on behalf of the American Thoracic Society ad hoc Committee on Healthy Sleep, "An Official American Thoracic Society Statement: The Importance of Healthy Sleep. Recommendations and Future Priorities," American Journal of Respiratory and Critical Care Medicine 191, no. 12 (June 15, 2015):1450–58. doi: 10.1164/rccm.201504-0767ST.

8. L. Besedovsky, T. Lange, and J. Born, "Sleep and immune function," *Pflügers Archive: European Journal of Physiology* 463, no. 1 (January 2012): 121–37. doi: 10.1007/s00424-011-1044-0.

9. Ramar et al., "Sleep is essential to health."

10. N. F. Watson, M. S. Badr, G. Belenky, et al., "Recommended Amount of Sleep for a Healthy Adult: A Joint Consensus Statement of the American Academy of Sleep Medicine and Sleep Research Society," *Sleep* 38, no. 6 June 1, 2015: 843–44. doi: 10.5665/sleep.4716.

11. E. C. Hammond and L. Garfinkel, "Coronary heart disease, stroke, and aortic aneurysm," *Archives of Environmental and Occupational Health* 19, no. 2 (August 1969): 167–82.

12. "2003 Sleep in America Poll," National Sleep Foundation, Washington, DC, 2003.

13. Kenneth D. Kochanek, Sherry L. Murphy, Jiaquan Xu, et al., "Mortality in the United States, 2013," NCHS data brief 178, no. 178 (2014): 1–8.

14. G. Stores, "Clinical diagnosis and misdiagnosis of sleep disorders," *Journal of Neurology, Neurosurgery and Psychiatry* 78, no 12 (December 2007): 1293–97. doi: 10.1136/jnnp.2006.111179.

15. M. Nagai, S. Hoshide, K. Kario, "Sleep duration as a risk factor for cardiovascular disease: A review of the recent literature," *Current Cardiology Reviews* 6, no. 1 (February 2010): 54–61. doi: 10.2174/157340310790231635.

16. D. J. Gottlieb, N. M. Punjabi, A. B. Newman, et al., "Association of sleep time with diabetes mellitus and impaired glucose tolerance," *Archives of Internal Medicine* 165, no. 8 (April 25, 2005): 863–67. doi: 10.1001/archinte.165.8.863.

17. K. Spiegel, R. Leproult, and E. Van Cauter, "Impact of sleep debt on metabolic and endocrine function," *Lancet* 354, no. 9188 (October 23, 1999): 1435–39. doi: 10.1016/S0140-6736(99)01376-8.

18. T. W. Kim, J. H. Jeong, S. C. Hong, "The impact of sleep and circadian disturbance on hormones and metabolism," *International Journal of Endocrinology* (March 2015): 591729. doi: 10.1155/2015/591729.

19. Ramar et al., "Sleep is essential to health."

20. S. S. Patterson, J. A. Kuchenbecker, J. R. Anderson, et al., "A Color Vision Circuit for Non-Image-Forming Vision in the Primate Retina," *Current Biology* 30, no. 7 (April 6, 2020): 1269–74.e2. doi: 10.1016/j.cub.2020.01.040.

21. S. Wahl, M. Engelhardt, P. Schaupp, "The inner clock: Blue light sets the human rhythm," *Journal of Biophotonics* 12, no. 12 (December 2019): e201900102. doi: 10.1002/jbio.201900102.

22. A. Charlot, F. Hutt, E. Sabatier, et al., "Beneficial Effects of Early Time-Restricted Feeding on Metabolic Diseases: Importance of Aligning Food Habits with the Circadian Clock," *Nutrients* 13, no. 5 (April 22, 2021): 1405. doi: 10.3390/nu13051405.

23. M. Geoffriau, J. Brun, G. Chazot et al., "The physiology and pharmacology of melatonin in humans," *Hormone Research* 49, no. 3–4 (1998): 136–41. doi: 10.1159/000023160.

24. "Melatonin: What You Need to Know," National Center for Complementary and Integrative Health, U.S. Department of Health and Human Services.

25. Geoffriau et al., "The physiology and pharmacology of melatonin in humans."

26. "CDC - How Much Sleep Do I Need? Sleep and Sleep," Centers for Disease Control and Prevention, March 2, 2017.

CHAPTER 6 HELP YOUR SELF STRESS LESS

1. "Stress," National Center for Complementary and Integrative Health, National Institutes of Health, April 2022, https://www.nccih.nih.gov/health/stress.

2. B. Chu, K. Marwaha, T. Sanvictores, et al., "Physiology, Stress Reaction," *StatPearls* (May 7, 2024).

3. G. Russell and S. Lightman, "The human stress response. *Nature Reviews Endocrinology* 15, no. 9 (September 2019): 525–34. doi: 10.1038/s41574-019-0228-0.

4. C. Jones and C. Gwenin, "Cortisol level dysregulation and its prevalence: Is it nature's alarm clock?," Physiological Reports 8, no. 24 (January 2021): e14644. doi: 10.14814/phy2.14644.

5. Jones and Gwenin, "Cortisol level dysregulation and its prevalence."

6. J. J. Kelly, G. Mangos, P. M. Williamson, et al., "Cortisol and hypertension," Clinical and Experimental Pharmacology and Physiology Supplement 25 (November 1998): S51–56. doi: 10.1111/j.1440-1681.1998.tb02301.x.

7. N. A. S. Mohd Azmi, N. Juliana, S. Azmani, et al., "Cortisol on Circadian Rhythm and Its Effect on Cardiovascular System," *International Journal of Environmental Research and Public Health* 18, no. 2 (January 14, 2021): 676. doi: 10.3390/ijerph18020676.

8. J. N. de Souza-Talarico, M. F. Marin, S. Sindi, et al., "Effects of stress hormones on the brain and cognition: Evidence from normal to pathological aging," Dementia & Neuropsychologia 5, no. 1 (January–March 2011): 8–16. doi: 10.1590/S1980-57642011DN05010003.

9. J. Rush, A. D. Ong, J. R. Piazza, et al., "Too little, too much, and 'just right': Exploring the 'goldilocks zone' of daily stress reactivity," *Emotion* 24, no. 5 (2024): 1249–58.

10. F. S. Dhabhar, "Effects of stress on immune function: the good, the bad, and the beautiful," *Immunologic Research* 58 (2014): 193–210.

11. A. Caplin, F. S. Chen, M. R. Beauchamp, et al., "The effects of exercise intensity on the cortisol response to a subsequent acute psychosocial

stressor," *Psychoneuroendocrinology* 131 (September 2021): 105336. https://doi.org/10.1016/j.psyneuen.2021.105336.

12. Y. Goto, S. Hayasaka, S. Kurihara, et al., "Physical and Mental Effects of Bathing: A Randomized Intervention Study," *Evidence-Based Complementary and Alternative Medicine* (June 7, 2018). https://doi.org/10.1155/2018/9521086.

13. Adrian L. Lopresti and Stephen J. Smith, "Ashwagandha (Withania somnifera) for the treatment and enhancement of mental and physical conditions: A systematic review of human trials," *Journal of Herbal Medicine* 28 (2021). https://doi.org/10.1016/j.hermed.2021.100434.

14. P. Jackson, J. Forster, J. Khan, et al., "Effects of Saffron Extract Supplementation on Mood, Well-Being, and Response to a Psychosocial Stressor in Healthy Adults: A Randomized, Double-Blind, Parallel Group, Clinical Trial," *Frontiers in Nutrition* 7 (2020). https://doi.org/10.3389/fnut.2020.606124.

15. Dhabhar, "Effects of stress on immune function."

16. Dhabhar, "Effects of stress on immune function."

17. S. Hidese, S. Ogawa, M. Ota, et al., "Effects of L-Theanine Administration on Stress-Related Symptoms and Cognitive Functions in Healthy Adults: A Randomized Controlled Trial," *Nutrients* 11, no. 10 (October 3, 2019): 2362. doi: 10.3390/nu11102362.

CHAPTER 7 HELP YOUR SELF
HAVE BETTER SEX

1. R. Swerdloff et al., "Sexual Function and Androgens," in Luciano Martini, ed., *Encyclopedia of Endocrine Diseases* (Academic Press, 2004).

2. D. A. Baribeau, E. Anagnostou, "Oxytocin and vasopressin: Linking pituitary neuropeptides and their receptors to social neurocircuits," *Frontiers in Neuroscience* 9 (September 2015): 335. doi: 10.3389/fnins.2015.00335.

3. S. Karama, A. R. Lecours, J. M Leroux, et al., "Areas of brain activation in males and females during viewing of erotic film excerpts," *Human Brain Mapping* 16, no. 1 (May 2002): 1–13. doi: 10.1002/hbm.10014.

4. "Autonomic Regulation of Sexual Function," in D. Purves, G. J. Augustine, D. Fitzpatrick, et al., eds., *Neuroscience*, 2nd ed. (Sinauer Associates; 2001), available at https://www.ncbi.nlm.nih.gov/books/NBK11157/.

5. P. Ueda, C. H. Mercer, and C. Ghaznavi, "Trends in Frequency of Sexual Activity and Number of Sexual Partners Among Adults Aged 18 to 44 Years in the US, 2000–2018," *JAMA Network Open* 3, no. 6 (June 1, 2020): e203833. doi: 10.1001/jamanetworkopen.2020.3833.

6. Z. Mei and D. Li, "The role of probiotics in vaginal health," *Frontiers in Cellular and Infectious Microbiology* 12 (July 28, 2022): 963868. doi: 10.3389/fcimb.2022.963868.

7. P. M. De Netto, K. F. Quek, and K. J. Golden, "Communication, the Heart of a Relationship: Examining Capitalization, Accommodation, and Self-Construal on Relationship Satisfaction," *Frontiers in Psychology* 12 (December 13, 2021): 767908. doi: 10.3389/fpsyg.2021.767908.

8. S. Gottlieb, "Frequent ejaculation may be linked to decreased risk of prostate cancer," *British Medical Journal* 328, no. 7444 (April 10, 2004): 851.

9. P. Haake, T. H. Krueger, and M. U. Goebel, "Effects of sexual arousal on lymphocyte subset circulation and cytokine production in man," *Neuroimmunomodulation* 11, no. 5 (2004): 293–98. doi: 10.1159/000079409.

10. M. Lastella, C. O'Mullan, J. L. Paterson, et al., "Sex and Sleep: Perceptions of Sex as a Sleep Promoting Behavior in the General Adult Population," *Frontiers in Public Health* 7 (March 4, 2019): 33. doi: 10.3389/fpubh.2019.00033.

11. S. Beerepoot, S. W. M. Luesken, M. Huisman, et al., "Enjoyment of Sexuality and Longevity in Late Midlife and Older Adults: The Longitudinal Ageing Study Amsterdam," *Journal of Applied Gerontology* 41, no. 6 (June 2022): 1615–24. doi: 10.1177/07334648221078852.

EDITOR
Rebecca Kaplan

DESIGNER
Kimberly Torgerson

CHART DESIGNS + ILLUSTRATIONS
Zoe Aniszfeld

MANAGING EDITOR
Lisa Silverman

PRODUCTION MANAGER
Sarah Masterson Hally

TEXT COPYRIGHT © 2025
Meredith Baird and Katerina Schneider

PHOTOGRAPHS COPYRIGHT © 2025
Haemi Lee

COVER © 2025
Abrams

Library of Congress Control Number:
2024936144

ISBN: 978-1-4197-7357-0
eISBN: 979-8-88707-277-7

Printed and bound in China
10 9 8 7 6 5 4 3 2 1

The medical information contained in
this book is not intended as a substitute
for the medical advice of physicians.
The publisher and author accept no
responsibility for any liability, loss or risk,
personal or otherwise, which is incurred
as a consequence, directly or indirectly
from the use and application of any of the
contents of this publication.

ABRAMS is represented in the UK and
Europe by Abrams & Chronicle Books,
1 West Smithfield, London EC1A 9JU
and Média-Participations, 57 rue Gaston
Tessier, 75166 Paris, France.
www.abramsandchronicle.co.uk and
www.media-participations.com
info@abramsandchronicle.co.uk

ABRAMS The Art of Books
195 Broadway, New York, NY 10007
abramsbooks.com